Enchanting Scents

D1489007

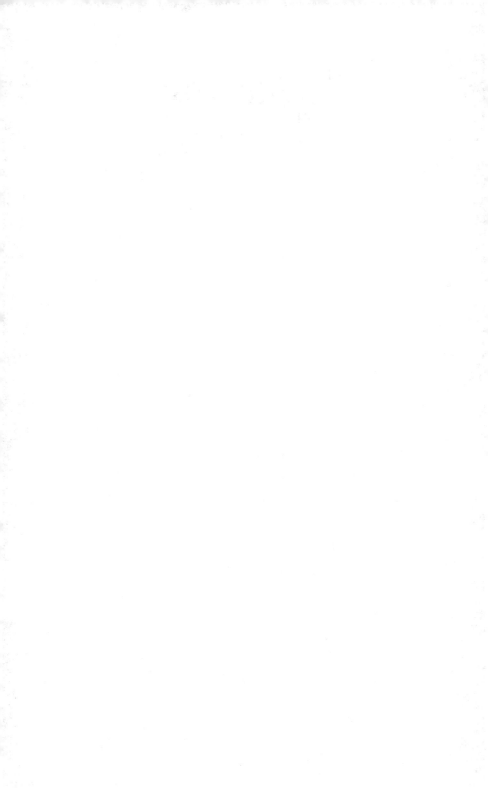

Monika Jünemann

Enchanting Scents

The Secrets of Aroma Therapy
Fragrant essences that stimulate,
activate and inspire
body, mind and spirit.

LOTUS LIGHT
SHANGRI-LA

1. American Edition 1988
by Lotus Light Publications
P. O. Box 2
Wilmot, WI 53192 U.S.A.
The Shangri-La series is published
in cooperation with Schneelöwe Verlagsberatung,
Federal Republic of Germany
Originally published 1988,
© by Schneelöwe Verlagsberatung,
Durach-Bechen, Federal Republic of Germany
Cover design and illustration: Wolfgang Jünemann
Illustrations by Martina Morlok
Translation and editing:
Christopher Baker and Judith Harrison, Munich
Editorial supervision: Monika Jünemann
Production: Schneelöwe, Durach-Bechen, Fed. Rep. of Germany
ISBN 0-941524-36-1

Printed 1988 in the Federal Republic of Germany

Contents

Introduction   9
Plants — A Link to Cosmic Consciousness   13
Essential Oils — The Essence of a Plant   17
The Nose — The Gateway to Consciousness   18
Breath — The Link Between Man and Nature   20
Essential Oils — Fragrances of a Special Kind   22

Essential Oils Described in Brief —   25
   (Origin, Production and Application)

Bergamot Oil 28, Cajeput Oil 29, Chamomile Oil 30,
Cinnamon Oil 31, Clary Oil 32, Clove Oil 33, Euca-
lyptus Oil 34, Fennel Oil 35, Frankincense Oil 35,
Geranium Oil 36, Ginger Oil 38, Jasmine Oil 39,
Juniper-Berry Oil 40, Lavender Oil 41, Lemon
Verbena Oil 42, Marjoram Oil 43, Mandarin Oil 44,
Neroli Oil 44, Niaouli Oil 45, Oregano Oil 46,
Patchouli Oil 47, Peppermint Oil 47, Rose Oil 48,
Rosemary Oil 49, Sage Oil 50, Sandalwood Oil 51,
Savory Oil 52, Thyme Oil 53, Vetiver Oil 54, Ylang-
Ylang Oil 55

The Use of Perfume Oil Lamps   57

The Soul of the Plant Touches the Soul of Man   58

Essential Oils — Energies of Transformation   60

Essential Oils for Promoting the Transformation
of Sensitivity and the Capacity for Feeling   65
  Lunar Energy   66
    Ylang-Ylang Oil   67
    Chamomile Oil   68
    Cinnamon Oil   69
    Clove Oil   70

Essential Oils for Promoting the Transformation
of the Faculty of Perception and
the Ability to Communicate   73
  Mercury Energy   74
    Lemon Verbena Oil   76
    Lavender Oil   77
    Savory Oil   78
    Peppermint Oil   79
    Fennel Oil   80
    Marjoram Oil   81

Essential Oils for Promoting the Transformation
of the Capacity to Relate and
the Ability to Love   83
  Venus Energy   84
    Rose Oil   86
    Sandalwood Oil   87
    Clary Oil   88
    Geranium Oil   90
    Ginger Oil   90

Essential Oils for Promoting the Transformation
of the Ability to Find One's Identity and
Take Action   93
  Solar Energy   94
    Bergamot Oil   95
    Neroli Oil   95
    Patchouli Oil   97
    Mandarin Oil   98

Essential Oils for Promoting the Transformation
of Willpower and the Will to Act   99
  Mars Energy   100
    Rosemary Oil   101
    Niaoli Oil   102
    Oregano Oil   103
    Sage Oil   104
    Thyme Oil   105

Essential Oils for Promoting the Transformation
of the Ability to Find the Meaning to Life   107
  Jupiter Energy   108
    Juniper Oil   109
    Vetiver Oil   110
    Jasmine Oil   111

Essential Oils for Promoting the Transformation
of the Ability to Concentrate   113
  Saturn Energy   114
    Frankincense Oil   115
    Eucalyptus Oil   116
    Cajeput Oil   117

Survey of Essential Oils and their Effects   118

Introduction

There are many excellent books about essential oils and aroma therapy, all containing information about the healing properties of aromatic oils and how they can be put to practical use. For example, many oils are indispensable in the treatment of a wide range of complaints, and since they act in an effective and swift-acting manner, I began to try them out on myself at one point. With time, my choice of oils became more and more exotic and they were soon replacing the allopathic and homeopathic remedies I had in my medicine cabinet. At the same time, I was slowly becoming more and more fascinated by their aromatic scent. The oils themselves healed my body, but on another level, their scent was affecting me in a way that I did not understand at the time. They seemed to alter both the mood I was in and the way I experienced reality. Despite this however, I was still primarily interested in the oils as a means of treatment.

Then, one day, a close friend of mine gave me a perfume oil lamp. I was soon making use of this extremely practical device in all kinds of situations, simply for pleasure. With time, I had perfume lamps in the bathroom, the bedroom and the office. These rooms all became the scene of much trial and experimentation with these delicate fragrances. Aroma therapy was becoming aroma magic.

Since I was guided by little other than my own interest in experimentation, the results were not always quite what I had been expecting. In one case, a long-awaited packet arrived one day, containing a bottle of clary oil which I had ordered from England since it was not obtainable in Germany in those days. As I happened to be in the office at the time, the first few drops of clary oil were sprinkled onto the perfume oil lamp we had standing there. It may well be that I sprinkled a few drops too many in my joy at getting the parcel, for what happened then was both pleasant and disastrous. Whatever the case, after a short while both my colleagues and I began to experience a cosy feeling of comfort and well-being which became quite euphoric for a while. This changed and gave way to a pleasant kind of laziness. We had a great time and did a lot of laughing, but we didn't get much work done. The following day wasn't as pleasant by far. This wasn't due to the clary oil, but to the mountain of work that had piled up in the meantime. As you can imagine, I never used clary oil in the office again, although I soon found situations where its effects were more welcome. Oils like geranium and savory are much better suited for the businesslike atmosphere of an office, for they aid concentration and promote activity.

It was during this time that I discovered that the use of perfumes to affect consciousness is as old as mankind itself. For thousands of years, man has liked to surround himself with aromatic perfumes and used essential oils to heal, relax, stimulate and intoxicate. It is no coincidence that religious ceremonies and rites of initiation are accompanied by the burning of incense. To this very day, the balsamic fragrance of frankincense is still associated with churches and holy places, for its scent appeals to all that in man that is susceptible to the transpersonal. On the other hand, no-one would think of using lavender or ylang-ylang in holy precincts, since these perfumes appeal too strongly to the sensual and physical side of man, as embodied by the lower energy centers or chakras. Indeed, ylang-ylang is made use in the treatment of impotence and frigidity, among other complaints, and is a component in perfumes that are said to have an aphrodisiac effect.

While there are certain occasions where the use of perfumes is deliberately avoided, there are others where essential oils, such as frankincense, rose or jasmine, are made use of out of a sense of tradition. Others again tend to reflect fashionable trends, such as patchouli, the perfume worn by the flower power generation during the 60's, and later on by all those wishing to open themselves up to the spirit of Eastern thought. I can still remember the smell of the Indian scarves that were so widespread at the beginning of the 70's. In those days, patchouli was a fragrance and label in one.

A fragrance can reawaken memories in us and give rise to many old associations, or it can send us off on paths of dream and fantasy. Perfumers who know how to use scents in this way are the master craftsmen of their trade. Many of them also use synthetic perfumes and animal substances, but since they have a very different vibration to pure essential oils, they are not to be discussed in this book. Only natural oils express the true essence of a plant.

Essential oils are extracted from plants growing in a dynamic energy field of earthly and cosmic vibrations. They represent something very valuable and precious which should be used with care and wisdom. This is one of the reasons why I have written this book, and this is what I mean by "aroma magic". Scents and smells influence our feelings and the way we react, whether we are aware of it or not. It is important to get to know the effects they have on us by watching how we react to them and getting to know the individual fragrances through and through. In this way, we can use them to the benefit of ourselves and others, for the conscious use of essential oils will help us on in our development and increase our sense of well-being. Essential oils mean joy — an immaterial yet substantial joy.

Plants – A Link to Cosmic Consciousness

It is hard to imagine life without plants. Indeed, as far as man as a species is concerned, they perform such important and extensive tasks that it is difficult to grasp their significance as a whole. For this reason, I would like to investigate what plants tell us about light, life and the plant world itself before turning to the individual fragrances in detail.

Life would not be possible on this planet – for us human beings at least – without water and air. Yet where does the air we breathe come from? There is only one elementary form of life that can communicate with man: the plant kingdom. Man and plants are interdependent, for each produces something that the other is in need of. In a pattern of give and take, plants produce oxygen and assimilate carbon dioxide and man produces carbon dioxide and consumes oxygen. These elementary processes are part of the great cycle in which every realm of nature takes up life in some shape and form and passes it on in another.

Life is contained in light, and light is solar energy. Without light, life would not be possible. We need light, but as human beings we cannot assimilate the vital energy it contains in a direct way. Were we to do so, we would literally burn up. We are only capable of taking in light, or solar energy, in the form of plant matter.

In plant life, the transformation of sunlight into energy is known as photosynthesis. Seen from a material point of view, energy is stored in plants in the form of sugars and starches, the fundamental constituents of our food. On a subtle level however, this is not all that takes place. With their roots in the soil and their leaves and blossoms reaching up towards the light, plants are capable of forming volatile, ethereal substances. With the help of the cosmic energy of light and the terrestrial energy of matter, plants are able to transform light into life. As already stated, light is a form of cosmic energy, and plants act as storehouses of this energy.

On a material level, we eat plants to nourish us and keep us alive, but we can only partake of their inner power, or essence, in another, more subtle way.

The knowledge that our ancestors had of the healing aspects of plants was not the result of long experimentation or analysis of active ingredients — indeed, these words did not even exist in those days — but was the consequence of their ability to communicate with the plants themselves. This is the only way in which man can partake of the life and essence of a plant. Devotion means giving of oneself unconditionally and it is only in the spirit of devotion that man can take and receive.

Communication with plants is an exchange in the consciousness of love, a balance of give and take which affects all dimensions of being. Plants are one of the forms of life which manifest cosmic consciousness on this earth and every plant we communicate with transmits this cosmic information to us.

However, communicating with plants does not necessarily mean talking to them. They can't audibly answer anyway. Here it implies a state of being aware and receptive. You could call it a meditative state of the highest alertness, a state in which you become totally receptive and in which consciousness can be truly experienced. Yet this is only one side of the coin. The spirit needs a counterpart in order to become manifest. It is the harmonious synthesis of matter and spirit which brings forth life as we know it.

Plants nourish us on a material level. By opening ourselves up to them, they also nurture us with cosmic energy. In this way, human consciousness can be regarded as a plant living within us that grows in accordance with our perception and consciousness of life.

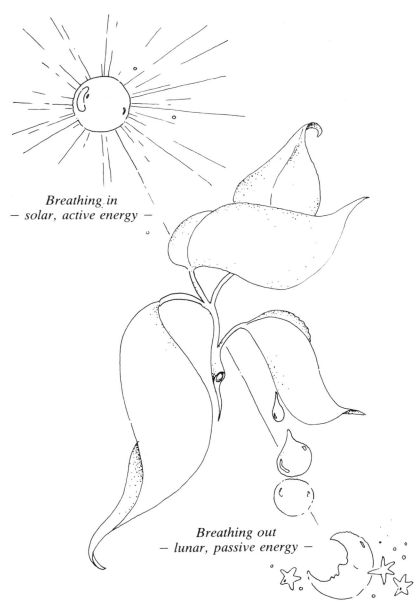

Breathing in
— solar, active energy —

Breathing out
— lunar, passive energy —

The plant, seen in the dynamic field
of polar life processes

Essential Oils –
The Essence of a Plant

Cosmic information is to be found in every part of a plant. In aromatic species this information is concentrated in certain volatile substances, otherwise known as essential oils or essences. An aromatic plant manifests its very essence in these ethereal oils, which are produced in small amounts and which volatilize according to the time of day and year and the positions of the stars.

In the human being, nerves transmit extremely fine impulses and glands secrete minimally small amounts of active substances in an involuntary and instinctual process that keeps the body alive. In plant life, the essential oils play a role that is comparable to that of the nervous and glandular system in man.

Essential oils are obtained by means of steam distillation, enfleurage, extraction and expression. Each oil is generally made up of differing constituents, but in many cases the exact composition is difficult to determine. But that isn't so very necessary. The main thing is that the oils exist and will continue to exist, since they are continually being produced by the plants in question. Due to the content of hydrocarbons, essential oils also exhibit volatile properties, that is, they tend to evaporate and become etheric. For this reason, they are also known as ethereal oils.

Ether is the primary matter of all life (according to

Greek philosophy), the bearer of life in the human body (according to Anthroposophy) or simply the energy of life (according to ayurvedic teachings). Ether, or life energy, is taken in by the nose, and for this reason, the nose is known as the gateway to human consciousness.

The Nose – The Gateway to Consciousness

With the very first breath it takes, the newborn infant enters an inseparable relationship with the energy of life. In India this energy is known as prana – and prana is taken in with the air we breathe. Western mysticism conveys this idea with the words, »And the Lord formed man out of a lump of mortal clay – and blew the living breath into his nose. And so man became a living soul«.

As ancient books state again and again – the fact that man lives is due to his relationship with this primary matter of life. The strength of a man's vital energy is dependent on the strength of this relationship.

Breath is the food of the soul. What we breathe and how we breathe it has a determining effect on our potential for creativity. The respiratory organs represent a means of influencing the control system of the subtle realms, otherwise known as consciousness. The nose itself is known as the gateway to human consciousness since it forms the directest link. Moreover, it is also the gateway of the sense of smell, the most differentiated and precise of all the senses. If the informational value of the sense of taste were to be compared to a magnifying-glass, the sense of smell would have to be equated to an electronic microscope. We can identify more smells than we can name.

The organ of smell, or olfaction, is located in the highest nasal convolution. You can only smell something when you breathe deeply, for only then does the breath pass over the olfactory field in which the olfactory receptors, or cilia, are located. The smells and prana inhaled with the air activate the cilia, which then transmit neural signals to the brain. (The exact way in which this process takes place is not entirely understood.) From here, further signals are transmitted via the spinal cord and the autonomic nervous system to every cell in the body. Olfactory impulses generally involve the so-called limbic lobe, a region of the brain which controls both emotions and memory. In contrast, the sensory perceptions of hearing and vision involve the thalamus, an area of the brain which only registers the simple sensations of warmth and pain. This explains why respiration and the perception of smell affect us in a deeper and more subtle way than all other forms of sensory perception.

With smell (breath), emotions and memory being so closely interwoven, the significance of pleasant-smelling fragrances becomes apparent, particularly in view of the fact that they can open up doors to the secrets of a deeper dimension of life.

Breath – the Link between Man and Nature

Beautiful fragrances awaken the desire in us to surrender ourselves to life. When we do this we open ourselves up to the cosmic rhythms of contraction and expansion in the natural interplay of inhalation and exhalation. The more fragrant a scent is, the better our respiration will be and the stronger our vital energy.

If vital energy is blocked, as it is when we are shocked and hold our breath, fear and tension result and we are no longer able to act to our full potential. If such a condition becomes an everyday event, our breathing becomes shallower and shorter as a result until finally the mind, body and soul fall ill due to the deficiency of prana. The same thing happens when we smell something unpleasant. In this case we avoid breathing deeply in order not to smell the unpleasant odor. As a result, our breathing becomes shallower. Our body is no longer provided with enough oxygen and our performance level sinks. In other words, exactly the opposite of what we want takes place. It is in this way that both body and psyche are made ill by a polluted and malodorous environment.

We all know that someone who does not breathe cannot stay alive. What we sometimes forget is that someone who does not breathe well does not live well either. When we smell something beautiful, our first impulse is breathe it in deeply. People seeking relaxa-

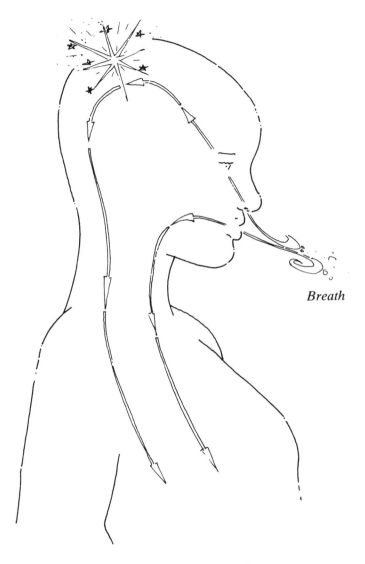

Life energy

Breath

The nose is the gateway to consciousness because
the energy of life is taken in with the air we breathe

tion and refreshment enjoy visiting fragrant woods, parks and gardens. A bouquet of flowers can mean an orgy of aromatic perfume. While nobody can rest or relax in badly-smelling surroundings, fragrant scents will lend wings to our imagination and awaken our zest for life.

Essential Oils – Fragrances of a Special Kind

The fragrances of essential oils are different to other kinds of pleasant smells and perfumes in that they consist of transformed solar energy. We can assimilate this energy with every breath we take and pervade our bodies with cosmic consciousness. It is no wonder that scents have always been put on a level with the divine and are often laid on altars in the form of an offering. While essential oils can be taken orally or massaged into the skin, they work best on a mental and spiritual level when breathed in through the nose. Indeed, it would seem that one of the tasks of essential oils on this earth is to be smelt – they almost seem to beg it. Perhaps this is the reason why they are endowed with the subtle and beautiful medium of scent.

Essential oils open up pathways to consciousness. Whether we notice it or not, or want it or not, smells, whether pleasant or not, can affect our moods and emotions. Our task is to find out as much as we can about the way scents affect us in order to apply this knowledge to our daily lives.

Through becoming aware of way fragrances can affect us, our faculties of perception and hence our experience of reality undergo an alchemistic process of transformation. Fragrances can release emotions and awaken joy. They can bewitch and soothe, inspire and liberate; they can take us back into the past, lead us on into the future or simply enchant us in the here and now.

Essential Oils Described in Brief

(Origin, Production and Application)

There are many different essential oils, but since only a few are of interest from a medical and commercial point of view, a lot of these are rare and consequently difficult to find. In my opinion, however, the range of natural essences generally available is large enough to allow for a certain amount of experimentation to be carried out, and so only a small selection is described. In each case, the oil in question is not only easily available, but has also proved to be of general interest and benefit.

Essential oils are to be found in all the parts of a plant, yet in many cases it has not yet been possible to determine where the oil is actually produced. Without our being able to say how this happens, it »suddenly« makes an appearance in the cell plasma and is then transported to certain storage organs. Both the content and transfer of oil to and from these organs is influenced by cosmic rhythms.

The main task of an essential oil is to organize the flow of information within the organism itself and to enable communication between the organism and other

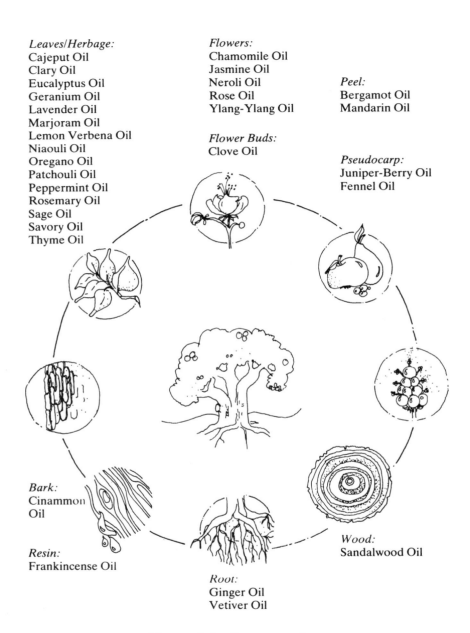

Leaves/Herbage:
Cajeput Oil
Clary Oil
Eucalyptus Oil
Geranium Oil
Lavender Oil
Marjoram Oil
Lemon Verbena Oil
Niaouli Oil
Oregano Oil
Patchouli Oil
Peppermint Oil
Rosemary Oil
Sage Oil
Savory Oil
Thyme Oil

Flowers:
Chamomile Oil
Jasmine Oil
Neroli Oil
Rose Oil
Ylang-Ylang Oil

Flower Buds:
Clove Oil

Peel:
Bergamot Oil
Mandarin Oil

Pseudocarp:
Juniper-Berry Oil
Fennel Oil

Bark:
Cinammon Oil

Resin:
Frankincense Oil

Wood:
Sandalwood Oil

Root:
Ginger Oil
Vetiver Oil

*Essential oils are to be
found in all parts of plants*

systems. Up to the present day, it has been discovered that essential oils
1. activate the metabolism of the system involved;
2. enable the exchange of information with microorganisms;
3. enable communication with neighboring plants;
4. repel potential enemies;
5. contain sexual attractants.

These characteristics closely resemble the ways in which we human beings put smells and fragrances to use, whether our own or in the form of perfume. With the help of essential oils, we can
1. activate the metabolism;
2. kill off bacteria and, with some species, repel insects;
3. signalize certain messages;
4. repel other organisms, such as bacteria and viruses;
5. stimulate our own sexuality and that of others.

In each of the five cases there is a very high possibility that the desired effect will be achieved, although this cannot be guaranteed to a 100 percent. For example, if someone can't stand the sight of you, none of the oils in the world will overcome this aversion. If there is a certain sympathy however, a touch of perfume oil will work wonders.

The best way to get to know a fragrance is via the nose. If you want to understand a scent in its wholeness, try to visualize the plant that produces it, growing and living in harmony with earthly and cosmic influences. Try and grasp its essence, for, like human beings, plants have an inner, invisible side as well as an outer, visible form, both expressing a single unity of being.

Bergamot Oil

The bergamot tree (Citrus bergamia) is chiefly cultivated in the high valleys of the south Italian province of Calabria, and in west India. The oil is extracted from the smooth-skinned, pear-shaped fruits, which resemble lemons in color, while they are still unripe. Due to its refreshing and sweet-smelling fragrance, the oil is indispensable to the cosmetic industry and it is one of the main constituents in eau de cologne. Since bergamot oil stimulates solar energy, it is has an animating and antidepressant effect. Bergamot oil belongs to the earth element group.

Cajeput Oil

The cajeput tree is a myrtle species that grows wild in Australia and Tasmania, where 90% of all species growing in the woods in this part of the world, including eucalyptus, are of the myrtle family. The cajeput, or paperbark, as it is also known, is an evergreen shrub with lanceolate, heather-like leaves and beautiful fragrant blossoms. The essential oil is obtained from several species of this plant, such as Melaleuca leucodendron and Melaleuca minor, which grows in Indonesia in the hot, damp climate of the Molucca islands, also known as the Spice islands. The acrid and pungent odor is slightly reminiscent of eucalyptus and turpentine. The oil is either colorless or with a yellow tinge, and is used in insect repellents and in the production of perfume. Due to its antispasmodic action, it is also used in natural healing for the treatment of complaints of the respiratory tract and the digestive system. Cajeput oil improves mental concentration and thus manifests the energy of Saturn. It belongs to the fire element group.

Chamomile Oil

Wild chamomile (Marticaria chamomilla) grows to about 12" in height. It has slender, pinnated leaves and a hollow and cone-shaped receptacle beneath the compact flower head. The white ray flowers bend downwards at night and when it rains. The chamomile will not grow on soil that has been treated with artificial fertilizer. Chamomile is mainly cultivated in the Balkan states, where it is grown over huge areas due to the demand. The essential oil is won from the flower-heads which are only harvested during bright sunshine because the content of essential oil sinks by half in misty and damp weather. The fresh, sweet-smelling fragrance of this greenish oil possesses lunar energy. Chamomile belongs to the fire element oil group.

Cinnamon Oil

Cinnamon oil is colorless and highly liquid and has a delicately fragrant aroma. The best oil is obtained by distilling the red-brown inner bark of the twigs of Cinnamomum zeylanicum, which grows in Ceylon. The cinnamon tree has small white flowers and oval opposite leaves which can grow to a length of about 4". The thin inner bark is also rolled into sticks for culinary use, and possesses the highest content of oil. Another, but less fragrant, version of cinnamon oil is distilled from the leaves, and is used in the production of soap, while the bark oil is employed in the creation of perfume. Most oils bought under the name of cinnamon oil are of the leaf variety. For example, Ceylon exported 70 tons of leaf oil in 1954, but only 176 pounds. of bark oil. Another kind of oil that is frequently sold under the name of cinnamon oil is the Chinese variety (Cinnamomum cassia or aromaticum), which is less fragrant than the oil produced in Ceylon.

Cinnamon oil possesses warm, lunar energy and belongs to the water element group.

Clary Oil

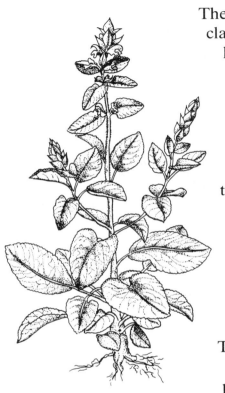

The Salvia sclarea variety of clary, or meadow sage, is a herbaceous annual which grows in Mediterranean countries on dry, rocky slopes. It is widely cultivated in Britain as a potherb and ornamental, and used to be grown in vineyards. The stalk is thickly covered with hairs and the grey, felt-like leaves are large and heart-shaped while the blossoms are small and a pale purple in color. The colorless oil, which is obtained from the whole plant, does not smell like medicinal sage, but has a distinctly sweet and fresh aroma of its own which is slightly reminiscent of lavender. Unlike lavender, however, clary oil does not activate the energy of Mercury, but rather the harmonious gracefulness and ease that is asso ciated with Venus. Clary oil belongs to the earth element group.

Clove Oil

Clove oil is expressed from the flower buds of Syzygium aromaticum before they burst into glorious red flower, since this is the time when they contain the highest amount of essential oil. The oil glands are located exactly below the epidermis of the ovary and contain about 18% essential oil, which is colorless when expressed. Syzygium aromaticum is an evergreen tree which can grow up to a height of 40'.

It is widely cultivated in the tropics, and grows in Africa, Central America, Malaysia and India. The pungent aroma is used in the production of perfume. Since clove oil is also used in dentistry because of its pain-relieving and antiseptic qualities, not every one will have it in the best of remembrance, particularly as it also used to be employed in an unpleasant-smelling insect repellant. But cloves also call pleasant memories to mind, such as apple pie and Christmas cookies. Whatever the case, we should not let ourselves be put off by the intensity of the smell or by unpleasant associations, for this pure and fragrant oil can be quite bewitching in diluted form. Clove oil possesses lunar energy and belongs to the earth element group.

Eucalyptus Oil

Eucalyptus oil, a colorless essential oil with an intense, camphor-like aroma, is mainly obtained from the leaves of the blue gum (Eucalyptus globulus), which is also known as the fever tree because of its excellent medicinal properties. There are about 600 varieties of eucalyptus (which belongs to the family of Myrtaceae), most of them growing in Australia. Eucalyptus trees can become very tall, the regnans variety reaching heights of up to 330'. The blue gum is a majestic tree with smooth, pale bark. The alternate blue-shimmering leaves take up a vertical position during hot periods to avoid the scorching heat of the sun and turn sideways at night to catch the falling dew. Another unusual characteristic of the eucalyptus tree is that its wood is heavier than water. Eucalyptus is indicated for fever and colds, both conditions in which it is not advisable to go out into the sun, and displays an antiseptic action that is higher than average. The oil also promotes the ability to learn from mistakes, thus manifesting the energy of Saturn. It belongs to the earth element group.

Fennel Oil

Fennel (Foeniculum vulgare) is a perennial herb that can take on magnificent proportions and reach a height of up to 4'.

It prefers a dry soil and is cultivated in temperate zones. The seeds are the part of the plant that contains the highest amount of essential oil and the scent is reminiscent of menthol and aniseed. South Indian varieties of fennel have a very low oil content. The oil is employed in natural healing to improve metabolic functioning and is known to be antispasmodic in effect, but can cause toxic reactions when taken in large doses. Fennel activates processes of intra- and extracellular exchange and thus can be seen as manifesting the Mercury principle. It also belongs to the air element group.

Frankincense Oil

Most people are familiar with the balsamic fragrance of frankincense from religious services. The scent is very difficult to describe, being aggressive and biting and yet gentle at the same time.

Frankincense is obtained from several species of the genus Burseraceae, the most important being Boswellia sacra, or incense tree, which is native to Africa and India.

Other Boswellia species also produce incense. The dried balsam is obtainable in granular form or in small pieces, but is generally not pure since it is mixed with other resins and substances.

Balsam is a resinous substance which is either stored in the tree in special cells, discharged into hollow cavities, or exuded onto the surface.

In most cases, an incision is made into the bark so that the resin can flow freely. Frankincense oil is colorless and highly liquid.

In old herbals it is indicated for practically every illness and complaint, but the main problem must have been the price.

Frankincense possesses solar and saturnine energy and belongs to the fire element group.

Geranium Oil

Geranium oil is obtained from a Pelargonium species belonging to the family of Geraniaceae. The wild geranium (which often has an unpleasantly pungent odor) has very little in common with the geraniums that are cultivated for the production of essential oil, and the potted geraniums of our homes and gardens are merely hybrids and not true geraniums.

Two Pelargonium species are of special interest in the production of the oil. One is the rose-pelargonium, (Pelargonium radula), a shrublike species with soft-wooded stems and palmated leaves, which is mainly cultivated in South Africa and in the mountainous regions of southern Europe. The leaves give off a rose-like scent at certain intervals and on touch. The oil is obtained from the whole plant by means of steam distillation, and is obtainable under the name of Reunion Oil (although it has nothing to do with the island of Réunion off the coast of South Africa) and "Rose Oil". The other species from which geranium oil is obtained is lemon-pelargonium (Pelargonium odorantissimum), which has a more lemon-like than rose-like scent, as the name would suggest. Both oils are popular ingredients in the production of soap and perfume, and are used for complaints of the lower abdomen, the skin and the kidneys in natural healing. Geranium oil has a harmonious effect. It possesses Venus energy and belongs to the earth element group.

Ginger Oil

The ginger plant looks like a small banana tree, and indeed, it belongs to a large family of banana-like plants which are mainly characterized by their potato-like tuberous rootstocks. The best-known species is Zingiber officinale, but Jamaica ginger, Bengal ginger and black (unpeeled) Barbados ginger, which produces a fragrant oil smelling of orange and jasmin, are also very popular. The oil of the Indian species of Zingiber cassumunar and Zingiber zerumbet is pale yellow and has a sweet-smelling, refreshing fragrance. Ginger oil is used in the production of liqueurs and sausage, and is employed as a herb in the treatment of indigestion, colds and rheumatism. It introduces an interesting and refreshing note to perfume mixtures. Ginger oil possesses Venus energy and belongs to the fire element group.

Jasmine Oil

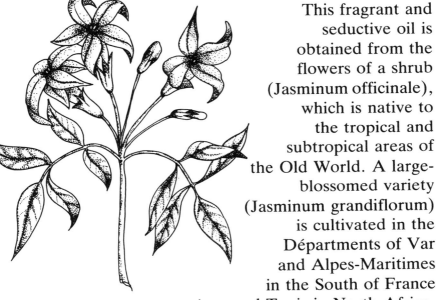

This fragrant and seductive oil is obtained from the flowers of a shrub (Jasminum officinale), which is native to the tropical and subtropical areas of the Old World. A large-blossomed variety (Jasminum grandiflorum) is cultivated in the Départments of Var and Alpes-Maritimes in the South of France and around Tunis in North Africa. Jasmine is also grown in Algeria, but here cultivation is restricted due to French over-production. The oil is obtained by enfleurage, a process in which the freshly picked flowers are laid onto layers of cold fat. The oil is extracted from the resulting pomade with alcohol or acetone and then purified. Perfumers take care to only buy oil that has been obtained gently from one kind of jasmine alone. »Huile antique au Jasmin« is a very popular variety which is obtained by sprinkling blossoms onto cloths soaked in olive oil, which are then wrung out. The copper-colored oil activates the warm and expansive qualities of Jupiter energy and belongs to the fire element group.

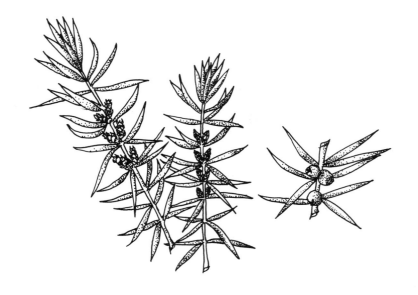

Juniper-Berry Oil

Despite the fact that juniper-berry oil is somewhat pungent, it is warm and relaxing in effect. The oil is obtained from the juniper tree (Juniperus communis), which is native to the whole of Europe, West Asia and North America. This robust and unpretentious shrub is to be found growing on poor soil at higher altitudes. A young juniper tree is long and slender, but when it gets old it branches out at the crown. The female inflorescences produce seed capsules in cone form which resemble berries. These berry-like cones are the parts of the plant that contain the essential oil. Juniper has always been a popular wood for fumigating and the essential oil is diuretic in effect. It possesses Jupiter energy and belongs to the water element group.

Lavender Oil

The genus of lavender (Lavandula) includes about three dozen species, all native to the Mediterranean and India. The essential oil is obtained from true lavender (Lavandula spika or Lavandula vera). The colorless oil, which has a stringent and refreshing character, has a rather »sedate« reputation. The thickly-growing shrub has greyish-green leaves which are slightly paler on the lower side. True lavender is cultivated in the South of France, but a more seldom variety is also grown in south England, and is highly esteemed. Lavender is particularly indicated for all disturbances accompanying nervous tension, and has a balancing effect. The oil can be employed in cases of palpitation, hysteria, spasmodic complaints of all kinds, sleeplessness, etc. Lavender soothes and calms the nerves and will stimulate the healing process, also in cases of outer injury. The speed with which this takes places indicates the Mercury character of the plant. Lavender oil belongs to the fire element group.

Lemon Verbena Oil

Lemon verbena (Aloysia triphylla) is cultivated in tropical and subtropical areas, where it also grows wild. It is a grasslike shrub with long, narrow, pointed leaves and small flowers. Due to its superb qualities, lemon verbena used to be a popular herb in natural healing, but it has now been largely forgotten. Lemon verbena oil has a clear, lemon-like fragrance. The oil possesses mercurial energy and belongs to the earth element group.

Marjoram Oil

The bushy perennial Marjorana hortensis originally came from West India, but it now grows all over Europe and is cultivated commercially around the Mediterranean. The colorless oil is obtained from the whole plant, including the square stems, the long leaves and the white labiated blossoms. The scent is reminiscent of a mixture of lemon and lavender. What is most striking about marjoram is that it has an anaphrodisiac effect, yet in spite of this, it is frequently employed in the production of perfume. Marjoram oil relaxes and alleviates tension, both mental and physical, and is used in natural healing for many complaints accompanying or caused by tension or a rigid way of thinking. This explains why it is seen to possess mercurial energy. Marjoram oil belongs to the air element group.

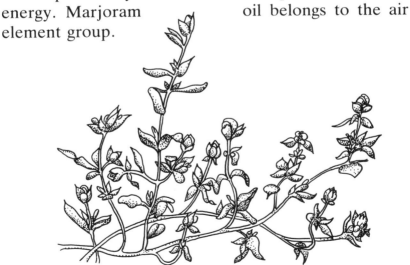

Mandarin Oil

The small mandarin tree (Citrus reticulata) is a native of China, but it is now also grown in south Italy and southern Spain, where the essential oil is produced in large amounts. The pale yellow oil has a fragrant, slightly bitter scent which is very popular in perfumery. Mandarin oil activates solar energy and belongs to the fire element group.

Neroli Oil

Neroli oil, which is obtained from the bitter orange tree (Citrus aurantinum) is one of the best-known oils and has an extremely feminine, fragrant aroma. The bitter, or Seville orange, is a sturdy tree which can reach a height of 16' to 50' and live to be very old. It can be seen growing in the Mediterranean, on the islands of the West Indies and in the Himalayas, where it grows on slopes facing south. The large white flowers of the bitter orange have an intense fragrant scent and the fruit has a rough-looking peel and tastes somewhat bitter. The colorless essential oil is obtained from the blossom, and is a fine and precious substance, much valued by the perfume industry. The peel also produces an oil, named bigarade oil (bigarade being the French word for bitter orange), which is comparable in quality to orange peel oil. Another oil, known as petitgrain, is obtained from the tender shoots and young oranges. Since the bitter orange is commercially cultivated in Spain, Sicily, South Africa and India, the fragrance can vary slightly according to origin. Neroli oil has the energy of the sun and belongs to the earth element group.

Niaouli Oil

Niaouli oil is obtained from a myrtle species named Melaleuca viridiflora, a close relation of Melaleuca leucodendron. The shrublike tree was discovered towards the end of the 18th century on the island of New Caledonia, where it grows profusely in the damp, warm climate. The colorless liquid oil has a stringent and acrid scent which is reminiscent of both peppermint and camphor. Niaouli oil activates Mars energy and belongs to the fire element group.

Oregano Oil

Oregano (Origanum heracleoticum) is a perennial herb that grows wild all over Europe. It can reach 1½' in height and has oval leaves and small mauve blossoms. The bitter and pungent odor of the pure oil is more reminiscent of old motor oil than of a fragrance that is valued by perfumers and soap-makers alike. Due to its content of essential oil, oregano is a popular culinary spice in Greece and other countries where generous use is made of oil. In this connection, it is interesting to note that oregano has recently been proved to possess properties that sink the level of cholesterol and lipids in the blood. While the gray-green oil can be used in a similar way to marjoram oil, it is classified as possessing Mars energy and as belonging to the fire element group.

Patchouli Oil

The patchouli (Pogostemon cablin) is a low shrubby mint cultivated in south and southeast Asia which belongs to the family of labiates. The brownish red oil is obtained from the long-stalked, oval leaves and is employed for medical purposes due to its antiseptic properties. However, its chief use is in the production of perfume, where it forms the basis of heavy exotic fragrances, lending them a »luxurious« touch. Alone, it has a heady, sweet-smelling aroma that is slightly musty at the same time. Patchouli oil possesses solar energy and belongs to the fire element group.

Peppermint Oil

Apart from central Africa and southeast Asia, the peppermint plant is to be found growing all over the world. Propagation is vegetative, via offshoots and runners that develop above and below the ground. The oil, which requires no description, is obtained from the oval, haircovered leaves of Mentha x piperita. Due to its high menthol content, it is used in most products that freshen the breath. In view of its lively and refreshing fragrance, it is no wonder that peppermint is seen as possessing mercurial energy and as belonging to the fire element group.

Rose Oil

Rose are grown all over the world in almost every garden, but the main area of commercial cultivation is still in Bulgaria, where the most exquisite and most expensive oil is distilled from the blossoms of the damask rose (Rosa damscena). Another rose oil is obtained in North Africa from the French rose (Rosa gallica). Since pure rose oil is prohibitively expensive, it is usually only available in diluted form. The fragrance of the greenish oil is unmistakable; it is the embodiment of perfume itself and is the most splendid of all essential oils. In natural healing, rose oil is employed in the treatment of complaints affecting menstruation and the lower abdomen, and is also used for skin care. It possess solar energy and belongs to the fire element group.

Rosemary Oil

Rosemary (Rosmarinus officinalis) is a fragrant ever-green shrub that can grow to about 6' in height. It is cultivated all over the Mediterranean and the essential oil is obtained from the leaves and blossoms by means of distillation and extraction. It has a refreshing and stimulating character and is used in natural healing for people who find it difficult to get going in the morning. It also stimulates the circulation and improves the supply of blood to all parts of the body. Rosemary oil possess Mars energy and belongs to the fire element group.

Sage Oil

True sage (Salvia officinalis) is a shrub that can reach a height of 1' to 2'. The leaves have a wonderful greyish-green tinge and the blossoms range from mauve to pink and purple in color. Sage likes a barren, often chalky soil in warm situations. The quality of the oil varies according to site and climate, as does the pungent scent, which is stronger in southern countries and milder when grown in the north. In large doses, sage oil can be toxic in effect. In diluted form it is used to lend aroma to wine and is employed in the cosmetic industry in the production of soap and mouthwash preparations. In natural healing it is used to treat inflammations of the mouth and throat area; it also has an antispasmodic effect and increases the blood pressure. Sage oil possesses Mars energy and belongs to the water element group.

Sandalwood Oil

The essential oil is obtained
from the heartwood of the
semi-parasitic sandalwood
tree (Santum album),
which is native to
Malaysia and the
Mysore district of
India. The tree has
evergreen opposite
leaves and
yellowish-gray
blossoms that
develop into
globular,
lemon-yellow
stone fruit. The
colorless, somewhat
sirupy oil has a fragrant
odor that, once smelt,
is never forgotten.
Sandalwood an excellent oil
for raising spirits. It possesses Venus energy and
belongs to the earth element group.

Savory Oil

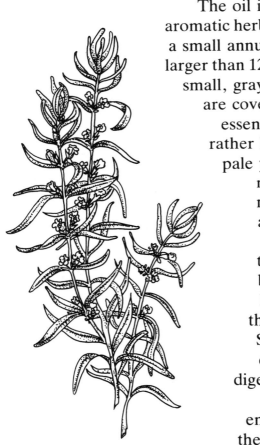

The oil is obtained from the aromatic herb Satureja hortensis, a small annual that rarely grows larger than 12". The stalk and the small, gray-green ovoid leaves are covered with hairs. The essential oil has an acrid, rather leathery odor and is pale yellow in color. It is mainly used as a culinary spice. Due to its aphrodisiac effect, it is sometimes added to sensual perfumes, but otherwise it finds little employment in the perfume industry. Savory oil stimulates cerebral activity and digestive functioning. It possesses Mercury energy and belongs to the fire element group.

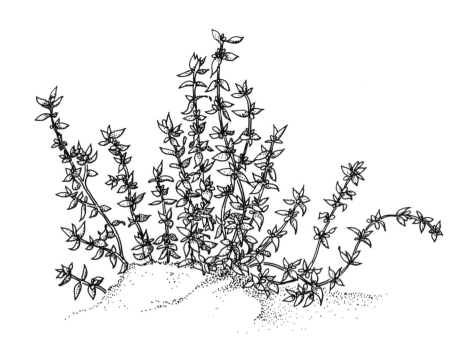

Thyme Oil

The colorless, highly liquid oil has an astringent and penetrating fragrance. Thymius vulgaris is a half shrub that reaches a height of about 7", and is a native of the Mediterranean, where it grows on rocky slopes and in the thick scrubby maquis typical of the region. While in natural healing, thyme oil is used externally for almost all complaints of the throat and chest, it finds little use in the perfume industry. Since flowery or sweet-smelling fragrances are not universally popular, it will lend a pungent and spicy note to oil mixtures for purifying the air. It possesses the energy of Mars and is an earth element oil.

Vetiver Oil

Vetiveria zinanioides (Andropogon muricatus) is a perennial grass native to Burma, Java, Indonesia and India, where it is also commercially cultivated. It is closely related to Zizania, the original rice plant. Vetiver grows in grass-like clumps and likes warm and moist soils. The brown to reddish-brown oil is highly liquid and is distilled from the roots, which are still dug out by hand and dried in the sun in some areas. The drying process is of some importance, for the care with which this is carried out is reflected in the quality of the oil, which should have a spicy, woody fragrance. The quality of the oil can also be affected by the methods of cultivation and processing. Other species, such as Andropogon squarrosus, citratus and nardus, are also cultivated for their essential oil. While it is rarely used in the West for medical purposes, vetiver oil is a popular remedy in India.

Vetiver oil is frequently employed in the creation of spicy perfumes. It activates Jupiter energy and is a fire element oil.

Ylang-Ylang Oil

Ylang-Ylang (Cananga odorata) is a subgenus of the annonaceae family, and is intensely cultivated in tropical regions. While other species of the same genus roduce essential oil of an excellent quality, they do so in tiny amounts, meaning that the oil available on the market is generally of the Cananga odorata variety. The pale yellow oil is distilled from the blossoms and has an unmistakable floral aroma. Indeed, ylang-ylang basically means "the fragrance of all fragrances" and is a firm favorite of the perfume industry, perhaps because of its aphrodisiac effect. Due to its sedative and anti-hypertensive action it is used in tonics, and is also employed as an additive in chewing-gum. It possesses lunar energy and is a water element oil.

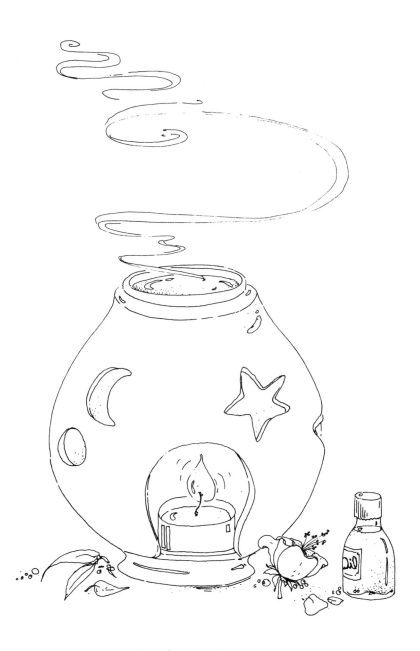

Perfume oil lamp

The Use of Perfume Oil Lamps

Essential oils are highly effective drugs. In small amounts they are antitoxic in effect, but in large doses they can be toxic. Instructions regarding length of use and strength of dosage must be followed to the letter when essential oils are taken internally (a form of treatment not described in this book.) Three to ten drops of oil sprinkled into a bowl of water will suffice to perfume a room the size of a fairly large bedroom; the exact dosage will depend on the volatility of the oil in question. For example, rose, geranium, ylang-ylang, jasmine, clary, neroli and frankincense can be dosed more sparingly than eucalyptus, rosemary, bergamot and chamomile. If too much perfumed air is inhaled, this can result in headache, nausea or other reactions, as listed below. An oral overdose of geranium will even result in death. However, you can be killed by too much of anything — it all depends on the amount. All the same, attention should be paid to the following contraindications.

Too long or too much inhalation of air perfumed with:

aniseed oil	can lead to a dazed feeling and, in some cases, nausea,
eucalyptus oil	can lead to nausea,
fennel oil	can lead to a dazed feeling; should not be inhaled when there is a predisposition to convulsive fits,
sage oil	can disrupt breast-feeding since it can obstruct the flow of milk,
thyme oil	can lead to profuse perspiration.

The Soul of the Plant Touches the Soul of Man

When we inhale an essential oil, it can profoundly effect our emotions, actions and reactions. Each essence has an unmistakable character, making it possible to place it into a group of other essential oils with a similar action. However, it cannot be claimed that all individuals will react in a certain, closely defined way, in the same way that we cannot say the same of the four temperaments, the signs of the zodiac, or the classification of people into personality types, such as introvert and extrovert. Useful and valid as these groupings may be, we have all experienced temperamental outbursts in otherwise introverted individuals or witnessed an energetic person of sanguine temperament in a somewhat apathetic state.

While it is possible to classify scents and fragrances into certain groups, we must remain aware of the fact that it is not possible to determine the exact effect they will have on the person in question. For example, a stimulating essential oil such as clary will sometimes turn out to have exactly the opposite effect, depending on the amount inhaled and the individual condition of the person involved. In this respect, aroma therapy via the nose is comparable to thet ancient Indian method of natural healing known as Ayurveda, a system in which statements are made regarding the effects of certain foods and medicines within the context of their use in different individuals. Ayurveda has defined three basic constitutional types (Rajas, Tamas, Sattva), which rarely manifest in their pure form but as a mixture of differing shares or percentages. An individual's constitutional make-up can only be determined for a certain period of time, due to the fact that all persons are subject to a continuous process of change.

The same approach must be taken with essential oils. In each case, we must take into consideration how we, or the person involved, is feeling at the time. Then, with the help of these oils, we have the possibility to react to even temporary situations or moods in a specific and appropriate manner.

As far as the use of essential oils is concerned, we should, indeed we must, go ahead and try out them out for ourselves. This applies to the approach I took to the oils dealt with in this book. I tried them out, acquainted myself with the plants that produced them and listened to what others had to say. With time, I was able to develop an increasingly clear idea of the »character« of the oils in question, and certain relationships between the oils and specific body centers and mental and emotional states began to emerge. This is not to say however, that an oil like lemon verbena, which has the effect of promoting mental activity, will be of use to someone who can't stand the smell of it. In such a case, it will probably distract him and rob him of all inspiration and leave him feeling cross and discontented.

We should always follow our nose in choosing an oil. It will soon tell us, perhaps after some initial practice, whether we need the oil in question and whether it will have a beneficial, healing effect on mind and body.

Essential Oils –
Energies of Transformation

Essential oils contain the transformed energy of the sun and planets, and as such, are able to affect the different levels of consciousness within us which are related to certain essential powers and faculties. If these levels are visualized as lying above each other like chakras, no one level can be considered superior to the other. At the same time, if one level, or faculty, is blocked, all the other levels and faculties will be affected accordingly.

This implies that consciousness is like a plant that grows and thrives within us, depending on how we develop our inherent faculties and powers.

Consciousness is a form of energy, the energy of life. The only way to preserve this energy is to transform it. The more energy we have, the more we feel happy and fulfilled. Energy gives us the strength to realize what we want, while consciousness gives us the ability to decide on how to go about getting it. By becoming aware of the energy at our disposal we can change the world – or consciously refuse to do so.

Essential oils have an effect on us because they embody the principle of transformed energy. However, they consist of this energy in concentrated form, meaning that they cannot be used in their pure state. If undiluted essential oil is applied to the skin, the result will be none too pleasant, for the skin will become red and irritated. If oils are taken orally in this form, the reactions will be revulsion and even nausea, because the aroma is too intense and concentrated. However, when we let these oils evaporate and gently unfold their ethereal character, we will experience them as fragrant and charming scents, affecting our consciousness, the etheric side of our nature, in a highly subtle way.

Essential oils activate the following aspects of consciousness:
1) sensitivity and the capacity for feeling,
2) the faculty of perception and the ability to communicate,
3) the ability to relate and the ability to love,
4) the ability to find one's own identity and the ability to take action,
5) willpower, and the will to act,
6) the ability to discover a meaning to life, and
7) the ability to accept responsibility.

Sensitivity and the capacity for feeling are the first faculties a newborn baby makes use of. These are very basic faculties, for it is only when we are sensitive and able to feel that we are able to perceive. Being able to perceive awakens the desire to communicate. In turn, the ability to relate and the capability of love are fundamental preconditions for discovering identity, and it is only when we have achieved this that we are we truly capable of taking action and expressing our identity through conscious deeds. Action spurred on by our sense of ego alone will invariably lead to disappointment, demonstrating the necessity to discover meaning in all that we do. This in turn makes us willing and able to accept responsibility. This is the point at which the

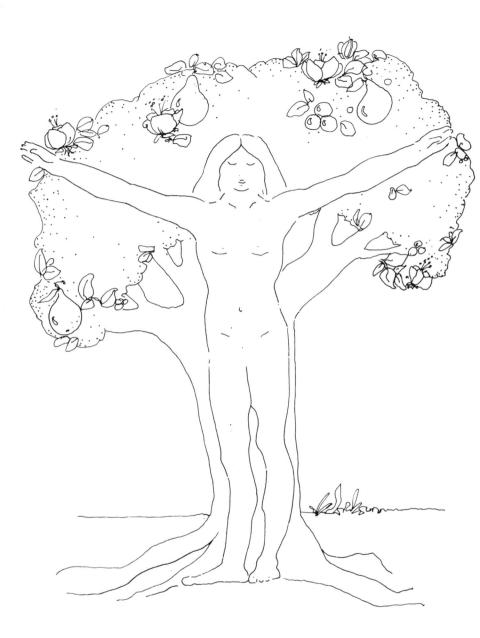

When we unite our consciousness with plants in love,
we open ourselves up to cosmic powers

circle is completed. From now on, any further progression will lead us up a spiral curve of development, for the more responsibility we accept, the more we will increase our sensitivity and capacity for feeling. The more we increase our sensitivity and capacity for feeling is increased, the more we will be able to perceive; the more we are able to perceive; the more ... Essential oils can become our companions on this spiral of development.

Essential Oils Promoting the Transformation of Sensitivity and the Capacity for Feeling

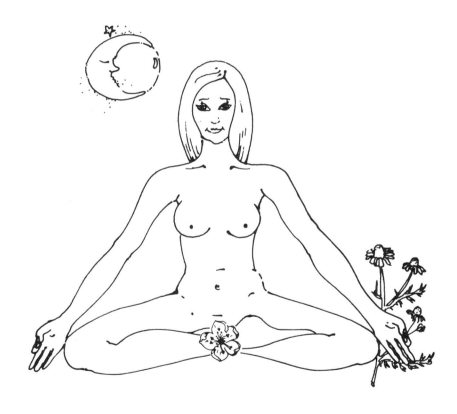

– Lunar Energy –

The first stage in this spiral corresponds to the ever-flowing energy of the moon. By surrounding ourselves with the fragrances of this energy form we give up a part of our individual personality and accept the principle of change. This includes all our feelings, which, like lunar energy itself, are continuously in a state of flux.

It is impossible to hold on to feelings and preserve them. All we can do is remember them.

Whenever we try to concentrate on a certain feeling, it will invariably lose something of its original intensity. The feeling of love for example, cannot be held tight but must be created every moment anew in order to stay alive. This the reason why we always want to be with the persons we love, or surround ourselves with beloved objects. Lunar fragrances entice us to devote ourselves entirely to the flow of life. They help us open ourselves up to the source of strength which lies in our unconscious and become more receptive to external impressions. Essential oils possessing lunar energy stimulate imagination and creativity – therefore we can make good use of their inspiring power when composing music, writing poetry or simply painting.

There are also moments in life when we are in danger of becoming overwhelmed by external impressions or the contents of our subconscious, moments when we feel the ground slipping away beneath our feet. If these impressions are not digested properly, they may give rise to panic and confusion. This is when we are faced with the dark aspects of lunar energy. In such a state we can easily fall prey to our every mood, and not recognizing the transitory nature of our feelings, find it hard to make decisions. In such a situation, lunar fragrances can help us to recover a state of balance again.

Ylang-Ylang Oil

This light yellow oil with its wonderfully sweet aroma awakens feelings of safety and security and creates an atmosphere of familiarity, in which we are able to open up and let ourselves fall, sinking into a soft cloud, the wide maternal skirts of the archetypal Great Mother, as it were, where we can feel safe and protected from harm. In this state, we are able to let go of all tension. What had previously seemed to be a boundary and limitation suddenly turns into a beautiful stretch of open and inviting countryside.

When we are disappointed and angry, ylang-ylang oil helps pacify our feelings, for it makes us aware of our attachments, our rigid adherence to concepts and our spiritual narrow-mindedness. Ylang-ylang helps us become open again and more expansive, so that our anger may give way to feelings of sadness and tears may flow …

By transforming the energy of this oil, we enter a state of relaxation and experience the urge to give of ourselves to others, to love and to receive love. It is this pleasant state of relaxation which explains the aphrodisiac action of ylang-ylang, an oil which is so relaxing in effect that the results are sometimes euphoric. The exotic and sensual fragrance of ylang-ylang is excellent for use in baths and in the bedroom. Since it opens us up to the messages of the unconscious, it will also promote artistic inspiration.

Chamomile Oil

This light yellow to greenish oil has a fresh, slightly sweet fragrance and reminds us of home. For many people, it conveys a feeling of security because it is frequently first encountered in domestic surroundings. Chamomile oil is calming and relaxing in effect, like the atmosphere created by a loving and caring mother.

When we are upset, depressed or simply sad, chamomile oil will give us the feeling that there is indeed something that will calm us down and ease our inner pain, and that we can find this strength within us if we are only willing to become truly sensitive toward ourselves. Chamomile oil has a relaxing effect and calms the nerves while possessing a stimulating action at the same time. In the resulting atmosphere of alert tranquility, we are in a better state to thoroughly digest the cause of the upset. Therefore, chamomile is useful for individuals with oversensitive nerves. We only react with stress symptoms when we are confronted with more than we are able to handle. When we are calm and relaxed, we are able to face life again without having to react with defensive attitudes and symptoms of stress symptoms, such as an upset stomach. But even if the latter were to take place, chamomile oil would be the answer, for it is an effective remedy in digestive complaints.

Cinnamon Oil

Cinnamon oil possesses the warming and soothing energies which is called for whenever a person has become rigid with the cold. This is the right oil for the time of the year when winter reigns and fierce icy winds blow across the bare landscape, carrying off all that lacks the strength to withstand their penetrating energy. In such times we feel a strong need to withdraw to the shelter of our home or the warmth of a harmonious family life. In such times, cinnamon oil can create an atmosphere in which we are able to give and receive warmth ourselves.

For many people, the scent of cinnamon oil calls back childhood memories and the recollection of the feeling of joyous anticipation that pervaded them in the Advent season. Against the bare backdrop of a naked, snow-covered landscape, cinnamon oil can also inspire us to fathom the depths of our being, discover archetypal images and project them onto the outer world. Being exposed to the fragrance of cinnamon oil during sleep will also help call forth dream images long submerged in us. Cinnamon oil may also help us experience natural forces in the forms of fairies, either when we are asleep or when we are out for a walk in the countryside. On a physical level, cinnamon oil has an antispasmodic action and increases the activity of our forces of resistance. It warms the entire organism and promotes the circulation. The fragrance of cinnamon oil may also be sexually stimulating, but in a very gentle, subtle way which is very soft and feminine. Perhaps that is why perfumes with cinnamon oil are so popular with women. As a perfume, cinnamon combines particularly well with lemon or ginger oil.

Clove Oil

Of all the lunar fragrances, clove oil has the strongest relationship to the material level. In order to be truly great, inner strength, no matter how effective, must prevail in the most changing of external circumstances. The fragrance of this essential oil can help us learn that the things we have created and our views of life are subject to the law of change. The more we are able to let go of things without bitterness and the more we are able to open up towards new possibilities, the more inwardly peaceful we will become. Whatever it is we want to or are forced to let go of, whether a piece of furniture we have become attached to, a picture or just an article of clothing, clove oil will help us do so — thus creating the possibility for something to take the place of the article we have just parted ourselves from.

When we invest too much energy into holding onto certain thoughts, certain conditions of pain, particularly in the head area, may occur, reminding us of this in a painful way. Clove oil will be a help in such cases, relaxing our nerves and alleviating the pain. The pure oil has a very stringent smell and should therefore be combined with other oils. Bergamot, ginger, thyme, jasmin and frankincense are well-suited companions. One or two drops of clove oil are sufficient for use with perfume lamps.

Essential Oils for the Transformation of the Faculty of Perception and the Ability to Communicate

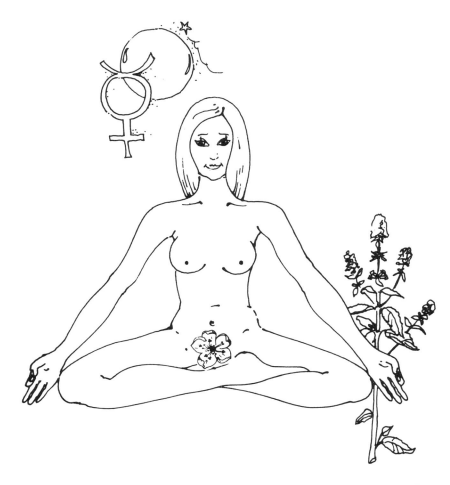

– Mercury Energy –

The energy of Mercury is quite unlike that of any other planet. It is not directed towards any particular goal or objective, but is more like a perpetual motion machine in that it serves the sole purpose of maintaining its self-generated energy. The energy of Mercury tolerates no standstill.

Mercury is devoted entirely to the task of transmitting information, whether within individual cells or between groups of them, whether between organ systems or throughout the entire organism, and in the exchange of information between mind, body and soul. As Mercury energy serves no other purpose than the flow and exchange of information, it has no inner mission or goals of its own that it need pursue.

Thus the essences which bear Mercury energy play the role of servants and transmitting agents. They act best in the rapid transmission of neural signals – in other words, in the areas of thought, communication and the exchange of information. They affect the speed at which transmission takes place, but not the informational content. A fast and efficient flow of information is always of great importance, for it helps us react adequately to the many different situations we are confronted with in life; it makes us tread on the brakes in time and find the right words on our lips, it helps us combine certain thoughts and come to certain conclusions.

On the other hand, all these functions need their necessary period of rest. The incessant desire to take action and the babble of never-ending trains of thought can be confusing and rob us of our strength. Instead of harnessing this form of energy for our benefit, we find ourselves at its prey. In such a state it might seem that our thoughts and actions are being determined by external circumstances, but it is we ourselves who have loosened the reins.

In pursuing our goals, developing our ideas and surveying our tasks, the oils of peppermint, lemon verbena and savory, which all manifest Mercury energy, will generally help to establish a smooth flow of ideas. Their action will assist us in finding the right words when writing and we may find that we are able to express ourselves more clearly and more concisely on the telephone. The efficiency of our office organization will be improved by the fragrances of these oils and conferences will run a better course. These oils can also be used to enhance creative work, and communication with others on these matters will also be facilitated by their use.

Fennel, lavender and marjoram will help us whenever we find ourselves being ruled by Mercury energy instead of commanding it as a servant. In such states, we are generally tortured by fixed ideas; torrents of thoughts keep us from finding peace and drive us on from one thing to another, like a train speeding across the open landscape. We have hardly taken note of one detail when we are on to the next, and then the one after it. Once Mercury energy is out of control, it seems impossible to bring it to a halt. We have no time to orient ourselves or change our hectic course. However, regaining tranquility is the only way to solve such a situation. In these cases, Mercury energy can only be overcome by Mercury energy. In this respect, lavender is a wonderful essential oil for inducing the deep relaxing sleep we need for analyzing our situation. Once we have slept a long night in this way, we will be able to differentiate between the positive and negative aspects of Mercury energy in the morning. Our mental clarity will increase and we will find life a lot more enjoyable.

Lemon Verbena

Lemon verbena's wonderfully light and refreshing, citrus-like fragrance makes it truly the king of the Mercury oils. It is unsurpassed in the acceleration of mental processes, as can be witnessed when we have been in a room scented with this oil. Although this fragrance does not exactly affect the actual process of producing ideas, it enables us to express them in a more concise manner. Lemon verbena is an ideal essential oil for the kind of people who have so many ideas and plans on their minds that they hardly know which one of them to pursue first. In times when a person is almost paralyzed by the endless possibilities or the wealth of tasks at hand, the fragrance of lemon verbena may prove to be exactly the right thing. It improves the capacity for deductive reasoning and thus enhances the pace of mental work. If we are planning a study trip, for example, we will be able to extract the best offers for our purposes out of a multitude of others in the shortest time possible, while determining the best travel route at the same time. It goes without saying that such a trip would not only include a visit to all the important sights, but would give us time to relax, and what is more, would be as economical as possible. This essential oil will help people who are striving for the highest degree of perfection to make the most out of their possibilities and potential.

Lavender Oil

If lemon verbena is the king of the Mercury oils, then lavender is the queen. Lemon verbena activates masculine energy and the principles of extroversion, dynamic action and light. Lavender possesses warming and relaxing qualities, and primarily affects the processes of communication within the organism itself. Lavender oil brings light to the shadowy aspects of Mercury energy: when our nervous system is agitated, over-excited and overwrought, the fragrance of lavender oil will help induce a state of welcome relaxation. When over-excitement is the cause of pain, lavender will alleviate and exert a soothing effect on mind, body and soul. When gnawing thoughts have caused us torturous headaches or cramped and painful shoulders, lavender will calm the cause of such complaints, namely the overwrought nervous system itself. The speed with which the message of "relaxation" is transmitted to all parts of the body manifests the Mercury character of lavender and is indeed truly amazing. When we find ourselves completely absorbed by worries and cares and are unable to let go of joyous or very sad events, lavender oil will prove to have a calming and soothing effect. Although lavender relaxes, it does not necessarily make us feel sleepy, but when sleep is necessary, it is an excellent tonic. Again, while it lends a lively and spicy note to perfume mixtures (one of the best known being eau de cologne), it spreads a rather Virgo-like atmosphere of cleanliness, pedantry and rational order when used alone. Unless used in the linen cupboard with the doors firmly closed, lavender is not the ideal oil for the bedroom. However, a combination of lavender and savory can prove to be quite arousing.

Savory Oil

The essential oil of savory has a soothing, relaxing action similar to that of lavender. Yet savory oil does not relax merely for the sake of establishing a state of relaxation but in order to create a balanced mood for launching new, innovative activities.

From a superficial point of view, savory does possess a certain relaxing effect, but basically, it is a very stimulating fragrance. One of the things it stimulates is the intellect. Difficult tasks become easier to deal with; if we have not been able to solve a complex mathematical problem, for example, the fragrance of savory may release the surge of mental energy necessary to solve the task at hand, despite the fact that we might have been on the verge of giving up. Savory oil activates the capacity for intellectual expression. This increase in performance efficiency not only manifests in the form of better cerebral functioning, it also affects our sexuality. Savory stimulates the desire for passion. Of course, this may not be what we need when dealing with mathematical problems, so it is important to pay attention to the point at which the fragrance begins to affect the lower energy centers instead of the upper ones. As an approximate guideline, three to four drops of savory oil in the perfume lamp will have a stimulating effect on cerebral functioning while a higher dosage will tend towards the opposite direction.

Peppermint Oil

If breath is the gateway to consciousness, then peppermint oil is an important key. This bracing, refreshing fragrance opens up the respiratory passages as no other oil does. Its cleansing and refreshing action on the respiratory tract and the channels of consciousness can be likened to a whirlwind. When our thoughts have reached a deadlock, our head feels heavy and we are fed up with things, a short deep whiff of peppermint oil will get us going again. We will suddenly regain interest in what we were doing and find that inspiration has returned to us. In natural healing, peppermint oil is used when such mental symptoms are caused by physical disorders.

Fennel Oil

Fennel is one of the feminine Mercury fragrances and activates maternal energy. For many people, the odor of fennel calls forth associations with childhood, of being cared for and protected by a loving mother.

Indeed, fennel has a particular affinity to mothers and small children, for it is useful in a multitude of minor complaints such as stomach-aches, coughs, running noses and light colds. This is due to its anti-spasmodic, carminative and germicidal action. Fennel is also an oil that promotes the formation of milk.

The fragrance of fennel encourages the desire to devote oneself entirely to a given task or person by giving of oneself unconditionally. The ability to perceive what others need is only possible when you are sensitive to your own needs. A person who knows how to be good towards him or herself will find it easier to genuinely help others. Only such people have the kind of courage necessary to do things that the other person may not understand or even be hurt by initially. Mothers in particular must be capable of acting with a certain loving firmness or strictness at times, even though it may cause them pain for a moment. In order for the personality to develop within certain limits, a child needs to experience the natural authority of the parents far more than the assurance of the ever-protecting parental hand hovering overhead. Here, the fragrance of fennel will prove to be a great help.

Marjoram Oil

Marjoram oil is one of the sedative, relaxing Mercury energy oils. Its stringent herbal fragrance envelopes us like a calming, sedating cloud which makes us want to close our eyes and take in the evaporating essence with all our senses. With every breath we take, we become more and more relaxed. The action of marjoram oil can be compared to being able to turn a little dial towards the "Off" position very, very slowly. This is just what we need whenever the inspiring power of Mercury energy threatens to turn into a state of nervous over-excitement, when we can't stop worrying and our thoughts go round and round and we become tense and rigid. Too much work and stress can also cause our mind and nervous system to become overwrought. When we have become agitated by hectic urban life, and are no longer able to digest a flood of impulses, when we are "fed up" with everything and no longer able to react adequately, marjoram oil is what we need to lead us back to a state of "hara" again. Once we are balanced and centered, we can consciously choose which influences we wish to expose ourselves to. On a physical level, marjoram oil stimulates digestive functioning and raises the sensory threshold of the organs of perception at the same time. Certain stimuli simply cease to call forth a reaction and we are able to concentrate on digesting what we have already experienced. Once this has taken place, we can open ourselves up to all that is new. The dulling, anaphrodisiac effect of marjoram on sexual desire is well known and indeed, sensory activity and sexuality are inseparably intertwined and mutually dependent; sexuality is sensuality. Thus a fragrance which has a sedative effect on sensory activity will invariably affect our sexuality.

Essential Oils for the Transformation of the Capacity to Relate and the Ability to Love

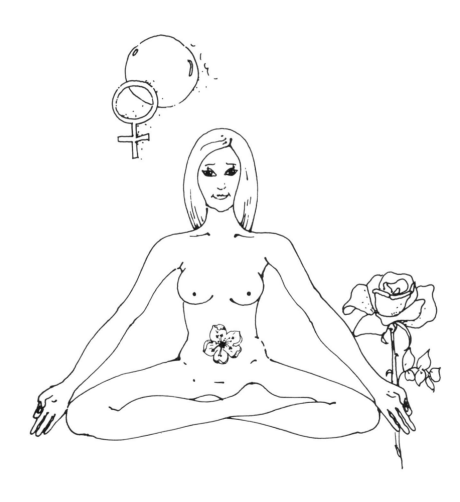

– Venus Energy –

These are essences possessing fragrances which correspond to the Venus principle, the irresistible urge to achieve harmony in all areas of life. The laws of harmony are inherent to nature. Harmony, however, can never be something static, but must always be found and created anew, again and again. Like the tone sequences in music, harmony is the directly perceived concordance of many individual components forming an integrated whole. A dualistic standpoint with concepts such as harmony and disharmony, heaven and hell etc., will not encourage our understanding of the dimensions of Venus energy. However, if we can imagine harmony as a principle occupying the center of a crystal ball, as it were (whereby our position is on the surface) it is clear that we can always be in touch with the central harmonious point no matter where we are on the surface of the ball and no matter the situation. This is why the astrological symbol of Venus consists of a circle, the symbol of holism, unity and spirituality, positioned above a cross, the symbol of matter. These two signs represent the union of spirit and matter, psyche and physis, life and death, sexuality and religion.

Inherent to Venus energy is the permanent challenge to find the center of one's personality, to mediate between one's own interests and those of the "others", to achieve a state of balance between technology and nature and to harmoniously unite sensuality and religion.

Essential oils which vibrate to this form of energy confront us with this challenge — each oil in its own specific manner and for a particular area of life. In each case, the task is always to establish a relationship between the inner and the outer world. The essence of harmony is basically the ability to love. It is expressed in the joy we experience when we pass on to others the impulses which we receive through plants and their fragrances, namely love and light.

Whatever it is that we love, whether a person or a certain goal, we will be able to attain it in the end. We will never be able to understand a person fully if we are not able to establish an open and loving relationship, and the same holds true for the fulfillment of any task we are faced with. We may come close to a goal, but we will never be able to achieve a state of unity with whatever it is we wish to attain — and this will be noticeable in the end, for ourselves as well as for others. When we fall short of our greatest potential, when we never empty the cup holding the water of life, our lives will always be lacking in an essential quality.

The fragrance of rose affects our relationship to sensuality and sexuality and the fragrance of geranium has an influence on our desire for justice, while the fragrance of ginger helps lend continuity to our thoughts and actions. Clary elevates our emotions to realms where freedom is just another word for having nothing left to lose, and sandalwood strengthens our bonds to spirituality.

Rose Oil

Joy, love, happiness, harmony, health, beauty and affluence — it would seem that all the desirable things in life can be associated with the enchanting scent of a rose. The rose is the most feminine and seductive fragrance of all the essential oils. On the one hand, it has an affect on the physical side of our nature and awakens the desire for sensual pleasures, such as delicious food, tastefully decorated surroundings, stimulating conversation and pleasurable physical contact. No wonder that lovers give each other roses. On the other hand, the fragrance of the rose touches our soul and transforms physical desire into the more subtle love for all sentient beings, for God and the transpersonal. This is the reason why temples were always adorned with roses.

The fragrance of the rose has the power to unite physical and spiritual love. Therefore the essence of rose was called "the blood of Venus" and placed under the protection of Aphrodite, the Goddess of love.

Rose oil is an aphrodisiac, yet it does not have the effect of arousing desire alone, for it instills this desire with the need for harmony, the need to find the partner one truly harmonizes with and the desire to establish a relationship possessing a very individual, personal balance between sexual pleasure and tender devotion.

The fragrance of rose transforms love into the art of love. Rose enhances the magic of human relationships and helps us experience them on all levels and depths of emotion, attaining a genuine synthesis between physical and spiritual love which is the source of beauty, joy and happiness.

The fragrance of rose oil is suitable for creating a private, intimate atmosphere as well as for use in public places such as offices, galleries and living rooms.

Sandalwood Oil

The fragrance of sandalwood oil is heavy and spicy and somewhat exotic.

Sandalwood oil has a strong affinity to man's urge to create. Whenever something is produced of timeless value, whenever concentrated spiritual power is expressed in ideas and works, we are able to experience the divine impulse of spiritual creativity – a power which reaches down into the depths of our innermost being and back through the aeons, enabling us to draw on the most ancient knowledge of mankind.

Sandalwood oil enhances our creative activity, for this unique fragrance stimulates the power of imagination; without imagination there would be neither ideas nor ideals. Imagination elevates our view of the world above and beyond our everyday cares and worries and lets us experience the realms of the spirit and fulfill our deepest yearning for love and realization.

The fragrance of sandalwood creates a feeling of happiness and joy, the feeling of creating something imperishable and of lasting value. This fragrance helps us liberate ourselves from the attachment to material, transient pleasures and to experience true inner contentment.

Sandalwood oil is a fragrance which can produce a euphoric state. At the same time, it also possesses a sedative action. It also has a sexually stimulating action which has been known and employed throughout the ages. In Buddhism and Hinduistic-Tantric practice, sandalwood oil is used as a stimulant, for it is felt that the sexual energy aroused by sandalwood oil can be transformed into certain states of consciousness and elevated to the pinnacle of spiritual experience.

It will certainly be rewarding to gather personal experience with the use of this essential oil.

Clary Oil

The sweet, refreshing fragrance of this oil is intoxicating. It is often experienced as a cloud that lifts you out of the everyday world, inducing a euphoric mood in which everything seems possible. Indeed, the fragrance of clary oil makes us aware of the limits set by consciousness and social convention and heightens our perception for ways and means of transcending these boundaries. Clary has the effect of encouraging us to take small steps beyond our familiar scope of action and thought. It awakens a pleasantly exciting desire to experience something new, the desire to discover the unknown inside us and experience its reflection in the outer world around us. Clary oil leads us into the depths of self-realization and self-knowledge and lets us experience the joy of spiritual transformation.

This process, which is basically what life is all about, can also lead to confusion, however, or be experienced as such. When attitudes or our view of the world change too abruptly, we can lose our balance and are no longer be firmly grounded − which is a basic precondition for taking substantial steps towards true personal change. Moreoever, if our rate of change is too rapid, the persons around us will not be able to follow us and we will find ourselves in a rather lonely position.

Clary is a most ambivalent fragrance. Finding the right dosage (less is more), is essential. Once we have managed this, we will be able to enjoy its positive effects to the full and go through any process of transformation at our own pace. Should headaches occur, it is wise to withdraw from this scent immediately. Two or three drops of clary oil in a perfume oil lamp are enough to create an atmosphere in which we may find relaxation, have inspiring thoughts or enjoy the warmth and tenderness of the one we love.

Geranium Oil

While clary is no oil for use in the office, geranium could be regarded as its counterpart, for it is out of place in the bedroom but all the better in the office.

The fragrance of this essential oil creates a refreshing, "public" atmosphere which will enhance the flow of conversation and facilitate the course of negotiations requiring a rapid, well-coordinated exchange of information.

With the help of the activating energy of this fragrance, we can find our natural rhythm, recognize our tasks and determine the sequence in which they must be dealt with. This is an essential oil which will instill all business dealings and activities with harmony and rhythm.

Ginger Oil

Ginger oil, which has an aromatic, refreshing fragrance, is a stimulating oil and a provider of energy. As it belongs to the category of Venus oils, it affects all activities concerned with the creation of esthetic and comfortable surroundings.

The way we chose to decorate and furnish our apartment, house or office is determined by our personal esthetic standards. This is a task which calls for clear decisions regarding to the coordination of individual factors such as the style of the furniture, the colors and materials used and the choice of accessory items. These factors have to be united into a harmonious whole in such a way that it is functional as well as meeting our esthetic standards. When we experience uncertainty in matters of esthetics and taste, the fragrance of ginger oil will help us make the right decisions.

The way we dress is an expression of our personal identity. When we lack the courage to try out something unconventional, a few drops of ginger perfume (50 drops of ginger oil to ½ fl. oz. of jojoba oil) may produce some astonishing results on the next shopping trip.

Essential Oils for the Transformation of the Ability to Find One's Identity and Take Action

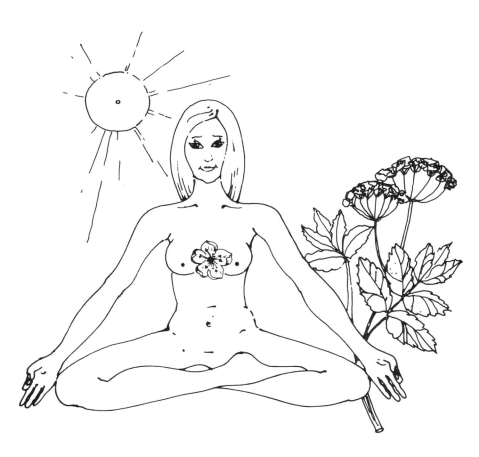

– Solar Energy –

The following essential oils activate the vital, life-affirming solar energy in us. By surrounding ourselves with these fragrances, we become aware of the fact that we possess a virtually inexhaustible source of energy that can be drawn on once we know what we want to do with our lives. When the goals we have set ourselves serve the development of our personality and lend expression to our solar essence, we experience solar energy as a light-bringing power. Our hearts open up to light, love and divine inspiration and become full of the joy of life and the desire to take action. Living our lives as intensely as possible and finding fulfillment in the here and now makes us warmhearted and truly capable of giving and receiving love. This energy can also be directed towards the objects which surround us and find expression in artistic and creative activity. There are no limits to the forms in which solar energy can find expression.

Bergamot, neroli and patchouli are the most potent essential oils possessing solar energy, and have proved to be excellent helpers in states of anxiety, fear and depression. Such conditions are characterized by an absence which occurs when we are no longer capable of absorbing the powers of light. Just as the light of the sun warms the earth and awakens a seed to life, letting it grow into a magnificent plant with beautiful flowers, it can also waken a similar seed within us and help it grow into a blossom of perfect beauty.

Bergamot Oil

Bergamot oil has a fresh and stimulating fragrance which affects our sense of being self-assured, the source of much of our life energy.

When we find ourselves in any kind of unfamiliar environment in which we feel unsure of ourselves, as during travel, this scent will help restore our sense of self-confidence. Again, when we have lost sight of the goals we are pursuing, the fragrance of bergamot oil will help clarify our objectives and lend us the strength to achieve our aims.

Whenever we find our plans darkened by the shadows of dark powers, this essential oil will help us focus a ray of concentrated light wherever it is most needed.

Neroli Oil

Neroli possesses the power of imbuing life with increased vitality, so that we no longer regard it from the standpoint of duties which must be fulfilled but regard it as a gift to be enjoyed to the utmost. Under the effect of this oil, our thoughts expand into a world beyond all limits. Neroli has a sweet, feminine odor which confirms our self-awareness and elevates us into a state in which we experience an endless desire for enterprise and action. Neroli is an expensive, luxurious oil with the strongest sedative and antidepressive action of all essential oils. What was previously inaccessible to us now seems to open itself up as if by magic, inviting us to enter a realm in which everything is possible — if only the immediate and honest expression of our inner essence. While neroli oil will help us overcome obstacles preventing us from achieving a healthy sense of self-confidence, it will not make us totally uninhibited in the process.

If we stay in a room perfumed with neroli oil for several hours, it will probably slow down our reactions, due to its sedative effect. For this reason, neroli is not an oil for use in the office and you should not use it when you have to drive. Like lavender, it is an excellent remedy for disturbed sleep. On the physical level, it is useful for all conditions involving excess tension and is also employed in the treatment of spasmodic and nervous heart complaints.

Patchouli Oil

This oil was the faithful companion of a whole generation in search of new forms of expression and new ways of finding one's identity — a generation in search of the meaning of life. This search found its expression in the ideals and symbols of the flower power movement — love and peace, unity and holism, meditation and music, flowers and beads. This fragrance embodies power, the power to walk down new and unconventional paths and become attuned to the rhythm of life. Having trodden the inner path of meditation, and having found the power of love within, the individual now seeks to make love and not war, in the widest sense of both words. The fragrance of patchouli also awakens a deep desire for peace. This extraordinary scent calls forth the desire to transcend inner and outer boundaries, to live and give of one's energy to the utmost in a spirit of all-encompassing love.

This is what makes patchouli oil such a unique stimulus for the act of love, for it arouses the desire to transcend all boundaries and enter into a state of total union with the beloved.

Mandarin Oil

The mandarin is the little sun of the heart. The oil has a gentle, mild yet refreshing fragrance and is most beneficial in helping us master the greyness of everyday life. While all chores which must be done day by day, month for month, year for year soon become more routine, they nevertheless offer us endless possibilities for lending expression to our capacity for taking action and can shore up our sense of identity. In fact, the sum of all these insignificant little everyday tasks amounts to a factor which has a much greater effect on us than our so-called "great goals" in life. And when we think about it, those great goals are only attained by taking an endless number of small steps.

The fragrance of mandarin oil can help us keep an open eye for these small steps and seemingly minor affairs. Others judge us by the way we deal with these minor details, and we ourselves can learn a lot through this means of self-recognition. Mandarin oil is an excellent fragrance for the Advent and winter season, and wonderful perfume mixtures can be created by mixing it with ylang-ylang, rose, jasmine and neroli. The effect of such a mixture will largely be determined by the oil most strongly present. We may find that a mixture of neroli and mandarin, for example, will help us direct our concepts and visions concerning what we wish to do and how we want to express it towards the small matters of everyday life. Feel free to experiment and discover the nuances that lie in other mixtures.

Essential Oils for the Transformation of Willpower and the Will to Act

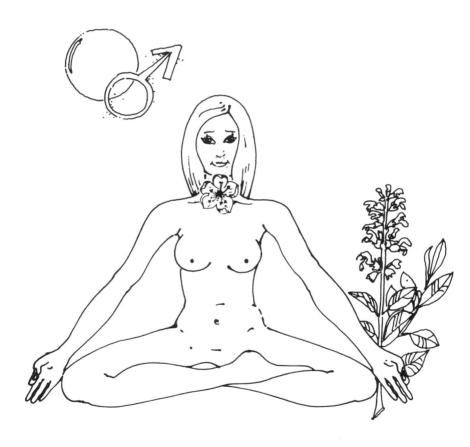

− Mars Energy −

There is no deed and no thought of a deed that does not cause a certain effect. Every deed, every thought of a deed, amounts to a tiny piece in the mosaic known as karma, and builds up a unique sequence of cause and effect. Whether we are aware of creating these causes or not, one day we will be confronted with their effects. Our life is the sum of many small actions and deeds and the direct and indirect effects they bring forth. Essential oils with a predominance of Mars energy act in two different ways. On the one hand, they may help bring unsteady and undirected activity to a halt, enabling the individual in question to find the clarity to refrain from such chaotic and thoughtless activity for a while and become composed enough to gather strength again.

On the other hand, these fragrances can also help in cases where there is too little energy or courage to realize one's goals in life. They can provide the necessary impulse to go beyond one's limits and do the impossible. They can also unlock considerable forces on an instinctual level.

Rosemary Oil

The essential oil of rosemary, which possesses a remarkably stringent and herbal fragrance with a hint of camphor, is one of the most stimulating of all the essential oils. On the physical level there seems to be nothing that cannot be activated by rosemary. It stimulates the functioning of the liver, the kidneys, the gallbladder and the heart as well as the female organs. This essential oil seems to cause every cell in the body to increase its rate of vibration.

When we inhale the fragrance of rosemary oil, something similar happens on a finer level, for our willpower and our willingness to act become extremely acute.

A few drops of rosemary oil in the bathtub or wash water in the morning will activate the energy we need for tackling what we have been planning to do on that particular day and will prevent us from falling prey to our inner laziness. Whatever we refrain from doing out of lack of motivation or weakness will always poison us in the end. By not accepting or admitting to our lethargy, we paralyze all further activity until the thing we initially sought to avoid has been dealt with. In such cases, the fragrance of rosemary oil will give us the strength to take the necessary steps, however difficult they may be. We are here on earth to be active and to take action. We have to organize our inner and outer lives in a satisfactory way, and that is hard work, but obstacles are there to be overcome.

Rosemary oil can be used when a certain problem causes us feelings of aversion which prevent us from taking action towards solving the difficulties involved right from the very start. Of course, not everyone has problems with this kind of thing — some people seem to be bursting with the spirit of enterprise — but there are many people who would be benefited by a few drops of rosemary oil and a few deeds accomplished.

Niaouli Oil

The essential oil of niaouli, which has a stringent, refreshing fragrance, affects the instinctual forces. In other words, it possesses transforming energies which have a particular affinity to sexual activity.

When two people meet who are sexually poled in opposite directions, as is normally, but not exclusively, the case between man and woman, and they feel sympathy for each other, and their "senders" and "receivers" are attuned to sexual vibrations, something may click between them and they will be drawn towards each other by the power of desire. When their bodies merge and melt into each other, desire can turn into joy, and physical lust and its gratification can become an expression of unconditional devotion which pervades mind, body and spirit. In a spirit of self-forgotten passion, the only desire is to give and experience the joy of union.

The essential oil of niaouli gives us the strength to restrain ourselves when predominantly physical urges seek their gratification. At the same time, it will also serve to enhance the erotic subtleties of love experienced in a physical union of joy.

Oregano Oil

The strong, bitter-pungent and somewhat dull fragrance of the essential oil of oregano is an excellent agent for removing us from the turbulence of everyday life in order to take stock of the energy we have left — particularly when physical and mental activities have left us in a somewhat depleted state.

Meditating in a room which has been scented with oregano oil will help us balance our energy household and come to grips with the tasks we still have to do. Due to its rather pungent smell, oregano oil is only suitable for short-term use.

Sage Oil

The essential oil of sage has a strong and activating fragrance and is fortifying and stimulating in effect.

The fresh essence has a particularly strong affinity to the respiratory tract and affects the strength of the voice. When we express what we want, we must not only speak the words physically, but also let them resonate in our soul. It is important for we ourselves to believe in what we say.

In order to be unequivocally understood, a clear intention must be expressed in equally clear and concise words. The tone of voice must be definite and should transmit strength and willpower. There are endless ways of saying "no". For example, a little girl reaches out to pull a tablecloth off the table. Her mother says "no", but at the same time, she remembers that she liked doing the same when she was a child. Despite the fact that the child hears "no", the subliminal message comes over with greater intensity. When confronted with such alternatives, a child will always pay more heed to the message which conforms to its own love for making discoveries. No wonder that many words are spoken without conveying their actual meaning, simply because they are not backed up by the right degree of determination. Sage helps lend strength and clarity to the human voice.

Thyme Oil

The energy of the essential oil of thyme has a stimulating effect on mind and body.

It is only through our actions that we are able to enter into relationship with the world and other people. It is only through our deeds that the power of creativity inherent to all human beings can be transformed into enlightened action — action in which it is possible to fulfil oneself by serving all sentient beings. In order to achieve this end, we need willpower, i. e. initiative, as well as courage and empathy. A fulfilled life is illuminated by the beauty inherent to acting in the right way.

As long as our actions are determined by envy, greed, fear or anger, we are on a path of confusion where we react to shadows instead of taking the initiative in a positive manner. When we pay attention to the effect of what we do in a spirit of conscious, loving devotion, our will is in accordance with the Divine Will. Once we have achieved this, we have also found the meaning to life, for we realize that the meaning to life is to overcome suffering and realize our own personal Shangri-La.

The essential oil of thyme strengthens us in the positive use of willpower, namely to manifest the will to be and the will to know in a conscious way.

Essential Oils for the Transformation of the Ability to Discover the Meaning to Life

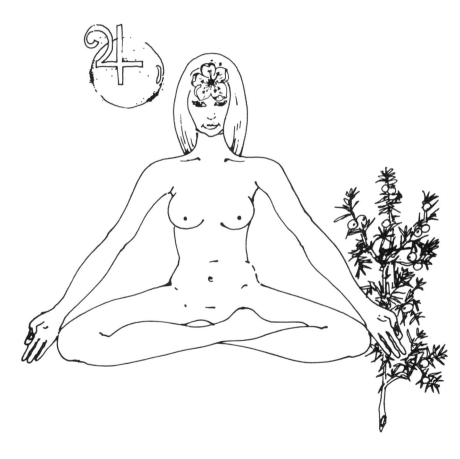

– Jupiter Energy –

The essential oils which represent the Jupiter principle lead us beyond the realms of everyday life. They have an affinity to areas which are situated almost entirely beyond all material bounds, but which are connected to them by a strong but silken thread.

The Jupiter principle is concerned with meaning, with the true meaning of the senses. Jupiter energy beckons us to recognize, interpret and realize the laws inherent to the rhythm of life and to come to an understanding of a transpersonal cosmic order. These essential oils stimulate our desire for initiation into a higher order of existence. This can express itself in a desire to discover what makes the world go round. We may set off on long journeys into untouched parts of nature or delve into the pulsating, decadent metropoles of our planet. The urge to discover the world can also be expressed in a deep interest in certain areas of knowledge. Time and space are no longer experienced as boundaries but as dimensions in which the mind may roam. The search for the meaning of life leads us to find our own ideals – ideals which can be found in the world of mundane events as well as in the world of the spirit. At the end of the search, we realize that all is indeed one, as the Taoists have always said.

When we use Jupiter oils, we no longer concern ourselves with the details and marginal aspects of life, but turn towards the unity of the cosmos, the transpersonal, the Divine, instead. Seen from this "pinnacle of realization" life begins to lose its tragic quality and the boundaries we normally experience as limitations gradually disappear, as we look over the hills and valleys of a never-ending expanse. We now regard the matters of everyday life with a degree of inner detachment and are aware of the duality of life with its ups and downs, coming and going, life and death. It is from this superordinate position that we can succeed in not identifying with the one or the other, but accept both aspects alike without losing our faith that are we indeed capable of changing the world.

Juniper-Berry Oil

When we have to meet the cold winds of reality head on with all our many little problems of everyday life, the stringent, spicy aroma of juniper-berry oil will help us gather the necessary inner strength to prevail amidst such difficulties and hold on to our higher ideals, even when our body is tired and threatens to drag our spirits down.

This essential oil has the effect of helping dissolve emotional attachments. On the physical level juniper-berry is a diuretic and helps rid the body of excess liquid. Its action on the psychological level is similar in that it helps us shed unwanted, "watery" emotions. This essential oil can be a great help in times when we find ourselves becoming too sentimental about things of the past and their negative emotional content. This is the case when we find that our journey on the path of realization is meeting with so many obstacles that we are losing sight of our guiding ideas and ideals. A juniper-berry perfume can be made by adding approximately 40 drops of essential juniper-berry oil to ¼ fl. oz. of jojoba oil. We can lightly massage a few drops of this mixture onto the bridge of the nose whenever we feel it might do us good.

Vetiver Oil

When we have succumbed to temptation and disregarded the guiding ideals of life and thus lost integrity, Vetiver oil will help us let go of false values and see what we really believe in.

The fragrance of vetiver oil awakens the desire to lead our lives in accordance with our highest ideals — we strive to realize the meaning of our life, to live according to the values we esteem, to attain wisdom and maintain an attitude of dignity in all situations in life. This can only be achieved by becoming truly idealistic and placing the needs of others above our own. Having realized the principle of ruling by serving, we find ourselves able to look far beyond the present moment and lead our lives in a spirit of tolerance and serenity. This oil will help us forgive our own shortcomings and those of others, and assist us in giving little thought and thus energy to temptations. In this way we will able to devote ourselves entirely to the higher goals we are pursuing in life.

Jasmine Oil

The sweet fragrance of jasmine oil arouses our spirits in very special way, beckoning us to phantasy worlds of lush, flowering meadows where we feel sensual yet as playful and care-free as a child. The action of this fragrance could be likened to a good and wise magician who can turn even the highest of our ideals into reality with a wave of his magic wand.

Jasmine also makes us receptive for temptations of all kinds. The sight of a certain flower may lead us into a world of memories or give rise to a yearning for things to come, a person we love may seduce us with tender caresses, or a certain thought may lead us off on long imaginary journeys to foreign countries or inner worlds.

The fragrance of jasmine invites us to relax and feel safe and secure, surrounded as we are by the laws of this and other worlds.

This unique fragrance may also arouse yearning for far-away places, the desire to set off on long journeys in discovery of foreign realms. Jasmine also has the affect of clearing away dark clouds of worry, for it is capable of leading us into a brighter world where life is worth living and where even the most melancholic of temperaments will be able see that life is also full of light and joy.

Essential Oils for the Transformation of the Power to Concentrate

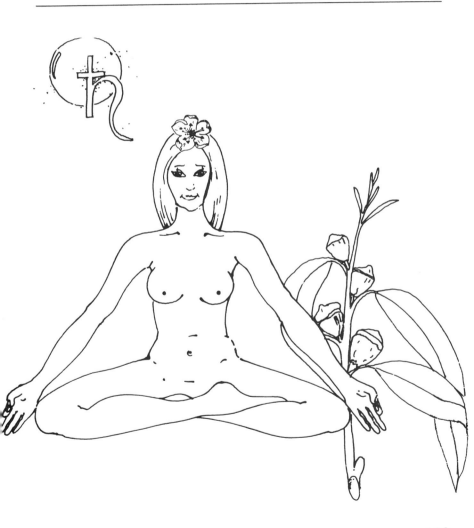

– Saturn Energy –

Essential oils which are carriers of saturnine energy help us learn to accept the limitations set by and necessary for life. The essential oils described so far give of their energy freely and place it entirely at the service of life. The saturnine essential oils are not concerned with giving energy but with preserving it instead. They are not oriented towards following the law of change governing the world of manifestation, but direct their energy towards all that is enduring, or permanent, within us and around us. By using these oils, we can practice the art of renunciation and cultivate the discipline of setting oneself necessary limits. This form of energy brings forth a healthy sense of ethics and morals. The realization of the laws of the world gives us the necessary strength to fight for what we have recognized as good and right, to delve deeply into the nature of things, to not succumb to the superficialities of the world, but to search for all that is enduring and protect it by erecting boundaries if necessary.

This is a tightrope walk between the positive and negative manifestations of saturnine energy and there is often only a thin dividing line between the healthy and necessary urge to find security, to cultivate reserve and the ability to be alone, and to search for what is lasting, on the one hand, and the negative aspects of this energy as evidenced by obstinate dogmatic persons whose fixed ideas concerning the preservation of life and values prevents them from living life at all.

Frankincense Oil

There are many people who may have an initial aversion to the fragrance of frankincense. This may be due to memories of times when the exuberant vitality of childhood was severely curbed by being forced to participate in religious ceremonies.

The fragrance and effect of the essential oil of frankincense are a great deal more subtle than that of frankincense burned on charcoal. This fragrance of the oil has a somewhat contradictory nature, but is also suitable for reconciling opposites. Since time immemorial, frankincense has been used in worship and rituals — its stern, heavy smell left man no doubt as to the transience of his existence and pointed towards paths to an eternal world which was more vaguely sensed than actually experienced. The fragrance of frankincense plays a mediating role between the gross material plane and more subtle levels by suppressing our instinctual and vital urges and stimulating our spiritual energy and our power of faith in a manner which is most extraordinary. This does not occur in a light, mercurial fashion, for a heavy saturnine hand forces us to acknowledge the laws of the cosmos and presses us to strive for realization and salvation. Used in small dosages, frankincense loses something of its heaviness and creates a balance between carnal desire and world-renouncing asceticism, reconciling as it were the opposites of red and blue into a gentle violet tone.

Eucalyptus Oil

Most people will be familiar with the fragrance of eucalyptus in the form of cough drops or other cough medicines. Eucalyptus has a very positive influence on the respiratory tract. The saturnine nature of this oil becomes very evident when it is inhaled. You get a feeling as if the air had got very heavy, and in stronger concentration the effect is oppressive and catches the breath. This also has its good sides, however, for there is hardly another essence which fills our lungs to such an extent and allows us to experience the significance of breath as eucalyptus does. The air we breath feels heavy — as if walking under eucalyptus trees shimmering in the summer heat — almost like breathing pure matter.

In less concentrated form eucalyptus is very good for all forms of breathing exercise and meditational breathing because it furthers the realization that we all breathe the same air, and are thus bound together and linked to all forms of sentient being. Eucalyptus can help us experience the transcendental dimension of these relationships.

Cajeput Oil

This fragrance reminds us of eucalyptus in a milder form. It imparts a feeling of safety and security which is rooted in the cultivation of tradition. Nothing can have a more confusing effect on our inner stability than breaking all too abruptly with what had previously provided us with security and continuity. Whenever the constancy of life has become upset due to our inability to realize the meaning of our duties and limitations, the fragrance of cajeput oil will be a valuable help. This scent helps create a meditative mood in which we are able to establish contact with the power from which constancy evolves. We are confronted with certain experiences in life again and again until we learn the lessons they have to teach us − and after every lesson we will be able to take a step beyond our previous limits.

Survey of Essential Oils and their Effects

Bergamot Oil
Scent: Fragrant, warm, with a touch of lemon
Energy: Sun
Element: Fire
Effect: Stimulating. Helps us trust in our senses; clarifies goals; activates light forces.

Cajeput Oil
Scent: Fresh, similar to eucalyptus
Energy: Saturn
Element: Fire
Effect: Balancing. Conveys a feeling of security; helps us take a constructive approach to life and learn from our experiences for the future; binds us to traditional values while helping us overcome them.

Chamomile Oil
Scent: Sweet, yet fresh and spicy at the same time
Energy: Moon
Element: Fire
Effect: Calming and relaxing. Brings about an inner sense of being balanced out and protected; soothes the nerves and stimulates physical and psychic digestion.

Cinnamon Oil
Scent: Warm and velvety
Energy: Moon
Element: Water
Effect: Relaxing. Conveys a feeling of warmth and protection; turns the attention inward; encourages dreaming and journeying into the world of the archetypal images of the soul.

Clary Oil
Scent: Sweet-smelling and fresh
Energy: Venus
Element: Earth
Effect: Relaxing and also intoxicating; widens our horizons and awakens our interest in things previously undreamt of; makes us undertake necessary changes in attitude.

Clove Oil
Scent: Stringent, extremely spicy
Energy: Moon
Element: Earth
Effect: Relaxes. Promotes willingness to let go of the old and the past and make room for the new. Particularly effects the material level.

Eucalyptus Oil
Scent: Refreshing, intense, with a touch of camphor
Energy: Saturn
Element: Earth
Effect: Balancing. Promotes respiration and is a good supporting measure for breathing exercises. Conveys a feeling of being united with all life.

Fennel Oil
Scent: Menthol-like, similar to aniseed
Energy: Mercury
Element: Air
Effect: Activates motherly energies. Gives us the strength to devote ourselves to the problems and troubles of others in a detached but loving manner.

Frankincense Oil
Scent: Balsamic
Energy: Saturn
Element: Fire
Effect: Harmonizing, mediates between the material world and subtle realms, suppresses instinctual energies and stimulates spiritual activity; strengthens belief.

Geranium Oil
Scent: Ranging from lemon- to rose-like
Energy: Venus
Element: Earth
Effect: Stimulating. Produces a fresh and open atmosphere; introduces an element of harmony and rhythm in our dealings with society; helps during talks and negotiations.

Ginger Oil
Scent: Sweet-smelling and refreshing
Energy: Venus
Element: Fire
Effect: Invigorating and harmonious. Useful in the creation of beautiful, esthetic surroundings.

Jasmine Oil
Scent: Fragrant and feminine
Energy: Jupiter
Element: Fire
Effect: Invigorating. Has a vitalizing effect and inspires us to discover new realms; promotes an effortless and lighthearted attitude and stimulates the imagination.

Juniper-Berry Oil
Scent: Stringent and spicy
Energy: Jupiter
Element: Fire
Effect: Balancing. Strengthens belief in ideas and ideals; clarifies the emotional sphere by literally washing away superfluous feelings.

Lavender Oil
Scent: Slightly stringent and bracing
Energy: Mercury
Element: Air
Effect: Warms and relaxes, calms down shaken feelings and alleviates tension and pain, both physical and mental.

Lemon Verbena Oil
Scent: Refreshing and lemon-like
Energy: Mercury
Element: Earth

Effect: Stimulating. Speeds up mental processes, heightens the power of concentration and mental acuity in general; helps achieve goals swiftly and effectively.

Marjoram Oil
Scent: Astringent and spicy
Energy: Mercury
Element: Air
Effect: Soothing. Lowers neural receptivity and raises the sensual threshold – also in sexual matters.

Mandarin Oil
Scent: Intense and with a flowery fragrance
Energy: Sun
Element: Fire
Effect: Balancing; helps get a grip on the routine aspects of everyday life and take action in small matters.

Neroli Oil
Scent: Refreshing, sweet and fragrant
Energy: Sun
Element: Earth
Effect. Extremely soothing. Promotes self-confidence and the ability to take the initiative and become more enterprising. Has an antidepressant effect.

Niaouli Oil
Scent: Stringent and fresh
Energy: Mars
Element: Fire
Effect: Stimulating. Activates sexual energy and arouses passion; makes you forget yourself and become more devoted.

Oregano Oil
Scent: Stringent and somewhat heavy
Energy: Mars
Element: Fire
Effect: Soothes and balances out; helps organize the energy at our disposal and put it to effective use.

Patchouli Oil
Scent: Fragrant and oriental
Energy: Sun
Element: Fire
Effect: Stimulating; provides us with the strength to follow unusual and individualistic paths; awakens the desire to transverse inner and outer boundaries.

Peppermint Oil
Scent: Fresh and menthol-like
Energy: Sun
Element: Fire
Effect: Stimulating. Clears the head and activates mental processes; awakens interest in one's surroundings.

Rose Oil
Scent: Fragrant and feminine
Energy: Sun
Element: Fire
Effect: Stimulating and seductive. Calls forth sensuality, which it transforms into an suprapersonal form of love. Cultivation of the art of love.

Rosemary Oil
Scent: Stringent and spicy, with a touch of camphor
Energy: Mars
Element: Fire
Effect: Stimulating, helps in cases of weakness and lack of drive; strengthens the willpower; promotes readiness to act and the ability to organize.

Sandalwood Oil
Scent: Sweet-scented and oriental
Energy: Venus
Element: Earth
Effect: Balancing. Has both a euphoric and soothing effect and stimulates the imagination. Inspires creative activity, initiates the transformation of sexual energy and awakens spiritual powers.

Sage Oil
Scent: Stringent and fresh
Energy: Mars
Element: Water
Effect: Stimulating; strengthens and clarifies the voice; has an invigorating effect in general.

Savory Oil
Scent: Stringent and leathery
Energy: Mercury
Element: Earth
Effect: Relaxing. Stimulates intellectual expressivity, but can also activate the sexual center when highly dosed.

Thyme Oil
Scent: Stringent and spicy
Energy: Mars
Element: Earth
Effect: Stimulates body and soul, confers courage, compassion and thirst for action, manifests the conscious will to be harnessed for the benefit of others.

Vetiver Oil
Scent: Acrid and wood-like
Energy: Jupiter
Element: Fire
Effect: Balancing; helps prevent being blinded by wrong ideas and promotes the realization of ideals. Also confers composure and tolerance and lends the strength to resist temptation.

Ylang-Ylang Oil
Scent: Sweet-smelling and fragrant
Energy: Moon
Element: Water
Effect: Relaxes, calms down feelings in cases of anger and disappointment, releases blocked feelings, stimulates the senses and has an aphrodisiac effect.

Angelika Höfler
I CHING
NEW SYSTEMS, METHODS
AND REVELATIONS
An innovative guide for all
of life's events and changes
190 Pages
ISBN 0-941524-37-X

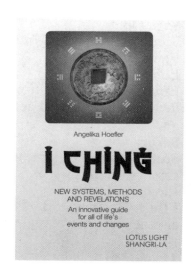

Angelika Hoefler

I CHING

NEW SYSTEMS, METHODS
AND REVELATIONS
An innovative guide
for all of life's
events and changes

LOTUS LIGHT
SHANGRI-LA

The I Ching – with new methods, new possibilities and new answers.

The author, herself actively interested in esoterics, studied characterology and applied as well as experimental psychology autodidactically, and has brought the eastern wisdom of the I Ching into poignant, contemporary language that includes glimpses of a knowing smile. In order to achieve exact answers, the hexagrams were divided into themes of inquiry, so that we can also receive concrete information about our own psychological make-up and condition, that of others and aspects of partnership. Each hexagram is accompanied by specific advice that is especially valuable in that it augments the partial as well as complete hexagram information, but can be applied independently of it. But the highlight of Angelika Hoefler's work is her development of a symbiosis of the I Ching and the Cabbala of Numbers, with which she has created a completely new system of cognition, of recognition and therewith practical help in life. We receive information. teachings, warnings, encouragement or advice, e. g. in questions of the right profession, place of education, living, work or vacation. Or in questions about the influence that certain persons or dates, agreements, names or titles to be decided on by us may have our success in life. Additionally, we gain clarity about where we stand in life—and this perhaps for the first time ever—what our functions and tasks are, where we belong and who belongs to us, and what the other person thinks about us.

Ursula Klinger-Raatz
THE SECRETS OF PRECIOUS
STONES
A Guide to the Activation of the
Seven Human Energy Centers,
Using Gemstones, Crystals and
Minerals
128 Pages
ISBN 0-941524-38-8

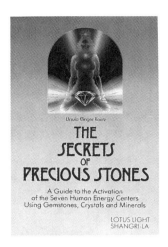

Ursula Klinger Raatz

THE
SECRETS
OF
PRECIOUS STONES

A Guide to the Activation
of the Seven Human Energy Centers
Using Gemstones, Crystals and Minerals

LOTUS LIGHT
SHANGRI-LA

Since time immemorial precious stones and crystals have been mysteriously fascinating for us human beings. Ursula Klinger Raatz describes the effects various stones have on our energy-body, which responds in a number of ways to the colors, qualities and uniqueness of minerals.

The author tells of her experiences with crystals and precious stones, describes the resonance they evoke, and explains how and why they are assigned to the different rainbow-colored energy centers of the human body.

This enables us to determine the healing vibrations of minerals right for us personally and to learn their practical application for the polarization of our energy centers, for healing using precious stones, and for entering into crystal meditation. Equally important, however, are the many impulses given for intuitive work with the secret powers inherent to the mineral world and particularly precious stones and crystals.

I CHING
New Systems, Methods, and Revelations

by Angelika Hoefler

$12.95; 185 pp.; paper; ISBN: 0-941524-37-X

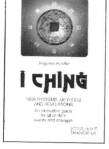

Innovative work on the I Ching, presenting new insights into the use of traditional forecasting tool, making it accessible to the modern reader. Beautifully designed including a meditation drawing for each Hexagram created by the British artist Terry Miller.

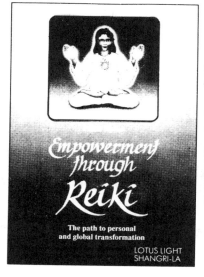

BESTSELLER:

Dr. Paula Horan
Empowerment Through Reiki

The path to personal and global transformation - a handbook

Length: 192 pages
Price: $14.95
Beautifully illustrated
Size: 18cm x 12 cm
ISBN: 0-941524-84-1

ENCHANTING SCENTS

by Monika Junemann

$9.95; 123 pp.; paper; ISBN: 941-524-36-1

The use of essential oils and fragant essences to stimulate, activate and inspire body, mind and spirit.

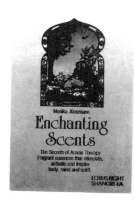

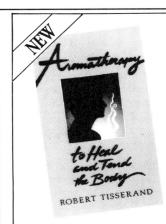
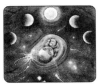
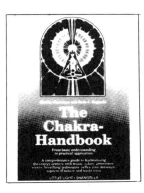

ADDRESSES and
SOURCES of SUPPLY
Fragrances, Gemstones, Herbs
Books and Cassettes

WHOLESALE

Contact with your business name,

resale number or practitioner license.

LOTUS LIGHT
Box 1008 ES
Silver Lake, WI 53170
Voice 414/889-8501 • Fax 414/889-8591

RETAIL

LOTUS FULFILLMENT SERVICE
33719 116th St, Box ES
Twin Lakes, WI 53181